Management of Cardiovascular Disease

Editor

DEBORAH L. WOLBRETTE

MEDICAL CLINICS OF NORTH AMERICA

www.medical.theclinics.com

Consulting Editors
DOUGLAS S. PAAUW
EDWARD R. BOLLARD

July 2015 • Volume 99 • Number 4

ELSEVIER

1600 John F. Kennedy Boulevard • Suite 1800 • Philadelphia, Pennsylvania, 19103-2899

http://www.theclinics.com

MEDICAL CLINICS OF NORTH AMERICA Volume 99, Number 4
July 2015 ISSN 0025-7125, ISBN-13: 978-0-323-39105-4

Editor: Jessica McCool
Developmental Editor: Susan Showalter

Medical Clinics of North America (ISSN 0025-7125) is published bimonthly by Elsevier Inc., 360 Park Avenue South, New York, NY 10010-1710. Months of publication are January, March, May, July, September, and November. Business and editorial offices: 1600 John F. Kennedy Boulevard, Suite 1800, Philadelphia, PA 19103-2899. Periodicals postage paid at New York, NY, and additional mailing offices. Subscription prices are USD $255.00 per year (US individuals), $471.00 per year (US institutions), $125.00 per year (US Students), $320.00 per year (Canadian individuals), $612.00 per year (Canadian institutions), $200.00 per year (Canadian and foreign students), $390.00 per year (foreign individuals), and $612.00 per year (foreign institutions). To receive student/resident rate, orders must be accompanied by name of affiliated institution, date of term, and the signature of program/residency coordinator on institution letterhead. Orders will be billed at individual rate until proof of status is received. Foreign air speed delivery is included in all Clinics' subscription prices. All prices are subject to change without notice. **POSTMASTER:** Send address changes to *Medical Clinics of North America*, Elsevier Health Sciences Division, Subscription Customer Service, 3251 Riverport Lane, Maryland Heights, MO 63043. **Customer Service: Telephone: 1-800-654-2452** (U.S. and Canada); **1-314-447-8871** (outside U.S. and Canada). **Fax: 314-447-8029. E-mail: journalscustomerserviceusa@elsevier.com** (for print support); **journalsonlinesupport-usa@elsevier.com** (for online support).

Reprints. For copies of 100 or more of articles in this publication, please contact the Commercial Reprints Department, Elsevier Inc., 360 Park Avenue South, New York, NY 10010-1710. Tel.: 212-633-3874; Fax: 212-633-3820; E-mail: reprints@elsevier.com.

Medical Clinics of North America is also published in Spanish by McGraw-Hill Interamericana Editores S. A., P.O. Box 5-237, 06500 Mexico, D.F., Mexico.

Medical Clinics of North America is covered in *MEDLINE/PubMed (Index Medicus), Current Contents, ASCA, Excerpta Medica, Science Citation Index,* and *ISI/BIOMED.*

PROGRAM OBJECTIVE

The goal of the *Medical Clinics of North America* is to keep practicing physicians up to date with current clinical practice by providing timely articles reviewing the state of the art in patient care.

TARGET AUDIENCE

All practicing physicians and other healthcare professionals.

LEARNING OBJECTIVES

Upon completion of this activity, participants will be able to:
1. Review the diagnosis and management of cardiovascular disease and high blood pressure.
2. Discuss treatment options for atrial fibrillation.
3. Recognize the use of technological advancements in monitoring the care of cardiac patients.

ACCREDITATION

The Elsevier Office of Continuing Medical Education (EOCME) is accredited by the Accreditation Council for Continuing Medical Education (ACCME) to provide continuing medical education for physicians.

The EOCME designates this enduring material for a maximum of 15 *AMA PRA Category 1 Credit*(s)™. Physicians should claim only the credit commensurate with the extent of their participation in the activity.

All other health care professionals requesting continuing education credit for this enduring material will be issued a certificate of participation.

DISCLOSURE OF CONFLICTS OF INTEREST

The EOCME assesses conflict of interest with its instructors, faculty, planners, and other individuals who are in a position to control the content of CME activities. All relevant conflicts of interest that are identified are thoroughly vetted by EOCME for fair balance, scientific objectivity, and patient care recommendations. EOCME is committed to providing its learners with CME activities that promote improvements or quality in healthcare and not a specific proprietary business or a commercial interest.

The planning committee, staff, authors and editors listed below have identified no financial relationships or relationships to products or devices they or their spouse/life partner have with commercial interest related to the content of this CME activity:

Wayne O. Adkisson, MD; Tariq Ali Ahmad, MD; Peter Alagona Jr, MD; David G Benditt, MD; Robert W.W. Biederman, MD, FACC, FAHA, FSGC, FASA; Edward R. Bollard, MD, DDS, FACP; Behnam Bozorgnia, MD; Blasé Carabello, MD, FACC; Umar Farooq, MD, MS; Sunita J. Ferns, MD, MRCPCH (UK); Lisa Filippone, MD; Anjali Fortna; Andrew J. Foy, MD; Paul J. Mather, MD, FACC, FACP; Jessica McCool; Talal Moukabary, MD; Gerald V. Naccarelli, MD, FACC, FHRS; Douglas S. Paauw, MD, MACP; Michael P. Pfeiffer, MD, FACC; Santha Priya; Sunita G. Ray, MD; Soraya M Samii, MD, PhD; Kunal Sarkar, MD; Mrinalini Sarkar, MD; Megan Suermann; Gian Paolo Ussia, MD; Deborah L. Wolbrette, MD.

The planning committee, staff, authors and editors listed below have identified financial relationships or relationships to products or devices they or their spouse/life partner have with commercial interest related to the content of this CME activity:

Javier E. Banchs, MD, FACC, FHRS is on the speakers' bureau for St. Jude Medical Inc., and is a consultant/advisor for Medtronic plc.

Mario D. Gonzalez, MD is on the speakers bureau for, a consultant/advisor for, and has research support from Biosense Webster, Inc.

David Lee Scher, MD, FACC, FHRS is on the speakers' bureau for Janssen Pharmaceuticals, Inc, and a consultant/advisor for Parallel 6; MedArchon Inc.; Frontline Medical Communications; Medscape, LLC.

UNAPPROVED/OFF-LABEL USE DISCLOSURE

The EOCME requires CME faculty to disclose to the participants:
1. When products or procedures being discussed are off-label, unlabelled, experimental, and/or investigational (not US Food and Drug Administration [FDA] approved); and
2. Any limitations on the information presented, such as data that are preliminary or that represent ongoing research, interim analyses, and/or unsupported opinions. Faculty may discuss information about pharmaceutical agents that is outside of FDA-approved labelling. This information is intended solely for CME and is not intended to promote off-label use of these medications. If you have any questions, contact the medical affairs department of the manufacturer for the most recent prescribing information.

TO ENROLL

To enroll in the *Medical Clinics of North America* Continuing Medical Education program, call customer service at 1-800-654-2452 or sign up online at http://www.theclinics.com/home/cme. The CME program is available to subscribers for an additional annual fee of USD $295.

METHOD OF PARTICIPATION

In order to claim credit, participants must complete the following:

1. Complete enrolment as indicated above.
2. Read the activity.
3. Complete the CME Test and Evaluation. Participants must achieve a score of 70% on the test. All CME Tests and Evaluations must be completed online.

CME INQUIRIES/SPECIAL NEEDS

For all CME inquiries or special needs, please contact elsevierCME@elsevier.com.

MEDICAL CLINICS OF NORTH AMERICA

THE CLINICS ARE AVAILABLE ONLINE!
Access your subscription at:
www.theclinics.com

Contributors

CONSULTING EDITORS

DOUGLAS S. PAAUW, MD, MACP
Professor of Medicine, Division of General Internal Medicine; Rathmann Family Foundation Endowed Chair for Patient-Centered Clinical Education, Medicine Student Programs, Professor of Medicine, University of Washington School of Medicine, Seattle, Washington

EDWARD R. BOLLARD, MD, DDS, FACP
Professor of Medicine, Associate Dean of Graduate Medical Education, Designated Institutional Official, Department of Medicine, Penn State–Hershey Medical Center/Penn State University College of Medicine, Hershey, Pennsylvania

EDITOR

DEBORAH L. WOLBRETTE, MD
Professor of Medicine, Penn State Milton S. Hershey Center, Penn State Hershey Heart and Vascular Institute, Hershey, Pennsylvania

AUTHORS

WAYNE O. ADKISSON, MD
Assistant Professor of Medicine, Cardiovascular Division, Cardiac Arrhythmia and Syncope Center, University of Minnesota Medical School, Minneapolis, Minnesota

TARIQ ALI AHMAD, MD
Assistant Professor of Medicine, Division of General Internal Medicine, Penn State Hershey Medical Center, Hershey, Pennsylvania

PETER ALAGONA Jr, MD
Program Director, Diagnostic Cardiology, Penn State Heart and Vascular Institute, Associate Professor of Medicine and Radiology, Penn State College of Medicine, Hershey, Pennsylvania

JAVIER E. BANCHS, MD, FACC, FHRS
Director of Electrophysiology and Pacing, Baylor Scott and White Health Central, Scott and White Memorial Hospital, Temple, Texas

DAVID G. BENDITT, MD
Professor of Medicine, Cardiovascular Division, Cardiac Arrhythmia and Syncope Center, University of Minnesota Medical School, Minneapolis, Minnesota

ROBERT W.W. BIEDERMAN, MD, FACC, FAHA, FSGC, FASA
Associate Professor of Medicine, Director, Cardiovascular Magnetic Resonance Imaging, Temple University School of Medicine; Allegheny General Hospital, Allegheny Health Network, Adjunct Associate Professor of Bioengineering, Carnegie Mellon University, Pittsburgh, Pennsylvania

BEHNAM BOZORGNIA, MD
Director, Advanced Heart Failure and Mechanical Circulatory Support, Einstein Medical Center, Philadelphia, Pennsylvania

BLASE CARABELLO, MD, FACC
Beth Israel Medical Center, Baird Hall, New York, New York

UMAR FAROOQ, MD, MS
Assistant Professor of Medicine, Division of Nephrology, Penn State College of Medicine, Hershey Medical Center, Hershey, Pennsylvania

SUNITA J. FERNS, MD, MRCPCH (UK)
Director, Pediatric Invasive Electrophysiology; Assistant Professor, Department of Pediatrics, University of North Carolina, College of Medicine, Chapel Hill, North Carolina

LISA FILIPPONE, MD
Assistant Professor, Department of Emergency Medicine, Cooper Medical School of Rowan University, Camden, New Jersey

ANDREW J. FOY, MD
Assistant Professor of Medicine and Public Health Sciences, Division of Cardiology, Heart and Vascular Institute, Milton S. Hershey Medical Center, Penn State University, Hershey, Pennsylvania

MARIO D. GONZALEZ, MD
Professor of Medicine, Director Clinical Electrophysiology, Penn State Heart and Vascular Institute, Milton S. Hershey Medical Center, Penn State University, Hershey, Pennsylvania

PAUL J. MATHER, MD, FACC, FACP
The Lubert Family Professor of Cardiology Director, Advanced Heart Failure and Cardiac Transplant Center, The Jefferson Heart Institute, Jefferson Medical College of Thomas Jefferson University, Philadelphia, Pennsylvania

TALAL MOUKABARY, MD
Clinical Electrophysiology, Penn State Heart and Vascular Institute, Milton S. Hershey Medical Center, Penn State University, Hershey, Pennsylvania

GERALD V. NACCARELLI, MD, FACC, FHRS
Professor of Medicine, Penn State Hershey Heart and Vascular Institute, Penn State College of Medicine, Hershey, Pennsylvania

MICHAEL P. PFEIFFER, MD, FACC
Assistant Professor of Medicine, Milton S. Hershey Medical Center, Penn State University, Hershey, Pennsylvania

SUNITA G. RAY, MD
Assistant Professor of Medicine, Division of Nephrology, Penn State College of Medicine, Hershey Medical Center, Hershey, Pennsylvania

SORAYA M. SAMII, MD, PhD
Associate Professor of Medicine, Penn State Hershey Heart and Vascular Institute, Milton S. Hershey Medical Center, Penn State University, Hershey, Pennsylvania

KUNAL SARKAR, MD
Department of Cardiology, Policlinico Tor Vergata, University of Rome, Rome, Italy

MRINALINI SARKAR, MD
Division of General Internal Medicine, Perelman School of Medicine, University of Pennsylvania, Philadelphia, Pennsylvania

DAVID LEE SCHER, MD, FACC, FHRS
Clinical Associate Professor of Medicine, Pennsylvania State College of Medicine, Hershey, Pennsylvania

GIAN PAOLO USSIA, MD
Department of Cardiology, Policlinico Tor Vergata, University of Rome, Rome, Italy

Contents

Syncope is one of several disorders that cause transient loss of consciousness. Cerebral hypoperfusion is the proximate cause of syncope. Transient or fixed autonomic nervous system dysfunction is a major contributor in many causes. A structured approach to the evaluation of syncope allows for more effective therapy.

Even after decades of progress in understanding atherosclerotic cardiovascular disease (ASCVD) and improved cardiovascular event prevention, the incidence, consequences and cost of cardiovascular disease (CVD) remain a significant public health issue. Observational studies have identified major ASCVD risk factors and lead to the development of a number of risk assessment systems/scores now in use. However many patients who will develop clinically important CVD are not identified by current systems or approaches and significant numbers of recurrent cardiovascular events continue to occur even after aggressive secondary prevention treatment strategies are utilized. Some now term this residual risk. The statin era revolutionized clinical practice with effective outcome-driven risk reduction. As a result there are now numerous clinical recommendations or guidelines for ASCVD risk stratification and treatment. Further disease and event prevention may rely on improved patient-centered risk stratification using novel biomarkers, imaging techniques, and new treatment approaches including emerging pharmacologic therapies.

The JNC 8 guidelines focus on 3 highest-ranked clinical questions that include BP thresholds for starting therapy, specific BP goals, and risks and benefits of specific antihypertensive drugs. Only randomized controlled trial data were used and JNC 8 panel did not include observational studies, systematic reviews, or meta-analyses. The investigators also suggested that benefit of lowering BP to less than 140/90 is not clear.

Lifestyle modifications were considered very important for all patients with hypertension. These recommendations are not alternatives for clinical judgment, and decisions about medical care must be individualized to each patient.

Valvular heart diseases (VHDs) place a hemodynamic load on the left and/or right ventricle that, if severe, prolonged, and untreated, damages the myocardium, leading to heart failure and death. Because all VHDs are mechanical problems, definitive therapy usually requires valve repair or replacement. In most valve disease the onset of symptoms marks a change in disease prognosis and is usually an indication for prompt surgical correction. Echocardiography is an indispensable modality for assessing lesion severity, its effect on cardiac function, and the proper timing for lesion correction. Intervention enhanced with percutaneous options now allows patients to benefit from mechanical correction.

Based on efficacy, safety, and ease of use, novel oral anticoagulants will likely replace VKAs for many if not most patients with atrial fibrillation. Novel anticoagulants have a lower rate of intracranial hemorrhage compared with vitamin K antagonists. The incidence of other life-threatening bleeds is similar if not lower. Dose adjustments need to be made based on renal function and advanced age. There is at present a need for an antidote for these new drugs.

Atrial fibrillation is a very common clinical problem with a high prevalence that is expected to rise over time because of increasing risk factors (eg, age, obesity, hypertension). This high prevalence is also associated with high cost, because atrial fibrillation represents about 1% of overall health care spending. The management of atrial fibrillation involves multiple facets: (1) management of underlying disease if present and the management of atrial fibrillation risk factors, (2) prevention of thromboembolism, (3) control of the ventricular rate during atrial fibrillation, and (4) restoration and maintenance of normal sinus rhythm.

Implantable cardiac devices are important management tools for patients with heart rhythm disorders and heart failure. In this article, the current implantable cardiac rhythm devices are described in their evolution. The current indications and contraindications for these cardiac rhythm devices are reviewed.

The advent of transcatheter aortic valve replacement (TAVR) has modified the treatment of severe aortic stenosis (AS). Large randomized trials and multicenter registries have endorsed the efficacy of TAVR in improving outcomes in patients with severe AS who are inoperable or high surgical risk. There has been a noticeable shift in using TAVR in patients with AS who are not at a high surgical risk. Appropriate diagnosis, patient selection, and referral remain cornerstones to achieving optimal outcomes after TAVR or SAVR (surgical aortic valve replacement).

Chest pain is a common complaint in the emergency department. Recognition of chest pain symptoms and electrocardiographic changes consistent with acute coronary syndrome (ACS) can lead to prompt initiation of goal-directed therapy. Cardiac troponin testing confirms the diagnosis of acute myocardial infarction, but does not reveal the mechanism of injury. When patients with chest pain rule out for ACS the use of advanced, noninvasive testing has not been found to be associated with better patient outcomes.

Cardiac magnetic resonance is well-established as a robust modality of cardiovascular imaging, providing superior resolution, infinite imaging planes, and the ability to obtain multiple types of information without ionizing radiation. Limitations imposed by availability, cost effectiveness, and safety prevent universal application. Many general and specialty practitioners do not have routine exposure to Cardiac MRI (CMR). Guidelines for the use of CMR exist, but continue to adapt to advances in techniques and ongoing research. Understanding the basics of CMR acquisition techniques, categories of appropriate use, and pertinent safety information will assist with selecting the best clinical scenarios to consider CMR.

Heart failure is a common syndrome caused by different abnormalities of the cardiovascular system that result in impairment of the ventricles in filling or ejecting blood. It is one of the most common causes of hospitalization in the United States, with a very high cost to the health care system. This article focuses on the causes of left ventricle dysfunction and the presentation and management of heart failure, both acute and chronic.

Current available mobile health technologies make possible earlier diagnosis and long-term monitoring of patients with cardiovascular diseases. Remote monitoring of patients with implantable devices and chronic diseases has resulted in better outcomes reducing health care costs and hospital admissions. New care models, which shift point of care to the outpatient setting and the patient's home, necessitate innovations in technology.

Foreword

Management of Cardiovascular Disease

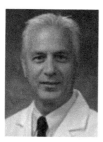

Edward R. Bollard, MD, DDS, FACP
Consulting Editor

Mortality due to cardiovascular disease in the United States has continued to decline over the last 15 years. Much of this is the result of incorporation of evidence-based guidelines in care, development of technology and new strategies to address these disease processes, as well as aggressive strategies for disease prevention as demonstrated in the most recent updates of the JNC 8 Guidelines for the Management of Hypertension in Adults as well as the ACC/AHA Guidelines on the Treatment of Blood Cholesterol to Reduce Atherosclerotic Cardiovascular Risk in Adults.

In this issue of *Medical Clinics of North America*, Dr Deborah Wolbrette has assembled a distinguished group of colleagues to present the most recent advances in the prevention, evaluation, and management of cardiovascular diseases and associated conditions. From the evaluation and management of syncope, the consideration and utilization of the new oral anticoagulant agents, to the patient selection and management of the transcatheter aortic valve replacement, these authors provide guidance to the practicing internist in the care of patients in a variety of both acute and chronic cardiac and vascular conditions.

Edward R. Bollard, MD, DDS, FACP
Department of Medicine
Penn State–Hershey Medical Center/
Penn State University College of Medicine
Hershey, PA 17033, USA

E-mail address:
ebollard@hmc.psu.edu

Med Clin N Am 99 (2015) xv
http://dx.doi.org/10.1016/j.mcna.2015.04.002
0025-7125/15/$ – see front matter © 2015 Published by Elsevier Inc.

Preface

CrossMark

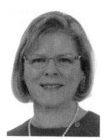

Deborah L. Wolbrette, MD
Editor

This issue of the *Medical Clinics of North America* provides an update of some of the more common and challenging management problems in cardiology. We are fortunate that our treatment of patients in many areas of cardiovascular medicine is founded on evidence-based guidelines. However, cardiology is a rapidly changing field. It is difficult to keep abreast of the new pharmacologic and interventional therapies as well as the evolving monitoring technologies. In many instances, the art of medicine is still needed to help navigate through the ever-changing guidelines and the sea of new modalities. The authors of this issue have tried to give the reader an expert perspective that the guidelines themselves cannot provide. The contributors have also concentrated on the key areas most needed by physicians outside of the field of cardiology.

This issue of the *Medical Clinics of North America* covers cardiac diagnoses commonly found in the primary care clinic, in the emergency department, or in the hospital. Atrial fibrillation is frequently seen in our aging population. Drs Moukabary and Gonzalez lay out very concisely the management of these patients. They very clearly outline the issues of anticoagulation risk and decisions of rate versus rhythm control. They also discuss the choice of antiarrhythmic drugs and who should be referred for ablation as well as ablation outcomes. The recent market release of the novel oral anticoagulants has provided a much needed alternative therapy to warfarin. The discussion by Drs Ferns and Naccarelli provides an excellent resource for the physician caring for patients on these drugs.

Heart failure is a frequent hospital admission diagnosis. In this issue, Drs Mather and Bozorgnia review the current recommendations for the acute and chronic management of heart failure. They also discuss when it is appropriate to refer to a heart failure specialist, and the role of hospice care. Chest pain is a common complaint encountered in the emergency department and many times presents a diagnostic challenge. Drs Foy and Fillippone have clarified some common misconceptions. After reading their evidence-based review, many readers will likely make some changes in their management of these patients.

Med Clin N Am 99 (2015) xvii–xviii
http://dx.doi.org/10.1016/j.mcna.2015.04.001
0025-7125/15/$ – see front matter © 2015 Published by Elsevier Inc.

medical.theclinics.com

We are most fortunate to have Dr Carabello discuss how to follow patients with mitral and aortic valve disease. He helps us understand the pathology of the lesion and how it relates to symptoms. He also helps clarify the decision-making process regarding the timing of surgery for these patients. Another group of challenging patients is those with syncope due to autonomic dysfunction. Drs Adkisson and Benditt give valuable clinical advice, helping us to avoid unnecessary testing. They also provide an understandable description of the different types of autonomic dysfunction.

Many primary care physicians are following patients with hypercholesterolemia and managing their lipid therapy. Drs Alagona and Ahmad provide an expert perspective on the available data and guidelines regarding cardiovascular risk assessment and prevention. They stress the need to assess and treat patients as individuals. Similarly, Drs Farooq and Ray discuss the latest guidelines for the management of hypertension.

Advances in technology have made a great impact on our diagnosis and management of cardiovascular disease. In interventional cardiology, transcatheter aortic valve replacement (TAVR) has provided an alternative to surgery for many high-risk patients with severe aortic stenosis. Drs Sarkar and Ussia describe the current landscape, the evolution of devices, and what the future holds for TAVR. In electrophysiology, remote monitoring capability allows home monitoring of patients with implanted devices as well as the ability to capture symptomatic arrhythmias. Drs Banchs and Scher discuss the progress that has been made so far in the digital technology field and give us a glimpse of what the future may hold in this area. Dr Samii reviews the current guidelines for implantable devices in a clear and concise manner. Cardiac MRI is a highly specialized imaging modality that continues to evolve. Drs Pfeiffer and Biederman provide information on the uses of cardiac MRI as well as a discussion of its limitations.

It is our hope that internists and cardiologists will find this issue of the *Medical Clinics of North America* useful in the management of patients in their practice. I would like to thank each of the authors for their contribution to the field of cardiology and their willingness to share their expertise with all of us.

Deborah L. Wolbrette, MD
Penn State Milton S. Hershey Center
Penn State Hershey Heart & Vascular Institute
Mail Code H047
500 University Drive
PO Box 850
Hershey, PA 17033-0850, USA

E-mail address:
dwolbrette@hmc.psu.edu

Syncope due to Autonomic Dysfunction

Diagnosis and Management

Wayne O. Adkisson, MD*, David G. Benditt, MD

KEYWORDS

- Syncope • Orthostatic hypotension • Primary and secondary autonomic dysfunction

KEY POINTS

- Syncope can result from any number of disorders that lead to transient self-terminating inadequate perfusion of the brain.
- A thorough and focused history is essential to arriving at the correct diagnosis; in many cases, a diagnosis can be reached without the need for additional testing.
- Patients with clearcut but rare episodes of reflex syncope (excluding carotid sinus syndrome) usually require no additional testing and no therapy beyond education and lifestyle modification.
- Syncope due to fixed or progressive autonomic nervous system (ANS) dysfunction is rare but is easily overlooked, often being dismissed as a simple fact of aging.
- Orthostatic hypotension due to fixed ANS dysfunction adds a significant burden to a patient already struggling with a neurologic disorder such as Parkinson or multisystem atrophy.

OBJECTIVES

The goal of this review is to offer a concise and practical review of syncope related to autonomic nervous system (ANS) failure and dysfunction. Syncope in the larger context of transient loss of consciousness (TLOC) is discussed briefly. This communication is not intended to be a comprehensive review of the diagnosis and management of syncope. For such, a review the European Society of Cardiology's 2009 guidelines is recommended.[1]

The primary objectives are to focus on the following:

- Conditions attributable to a failure of autonomic regulation, including
  - Reflex-mediated syndromes, including situational syncope, and
  - Primary and secondary ANS failure

Disclosures: None.

Cardiovascular Division, Cardiac Arrhythmia and Syncope Center, University of Minnesota Medical School, Minneapolis, MN 55455, USA

* Corresponding author. Mail Code 508, 420 Delaware Street South East, Minneapolis, MN 55455.

E-mail address: adki0004@umn.edu

Med Clin N Am 99 (2015) 691–710

http://dx.doi.org/10.1016/j.mcna.2015.02.002

medical.theclinics.com

- Clinical recognition and management of common syncope syndromes associated with autonomic dysfunction
- Essential diagnostic testing and avoidance of commonly ordered studies that are of little or no clinical utility.

INTRODUCTION

Syncope is one of several disorders included in the more general category of TLOC (**Fig. 1**). An obligatory feature of the definition of syncope is loss of consciousness (LOC); without LOC, by definition, syncope has not occurred. Furthermore, syncope episodes are transient (usually <1 minute) and resolve without need for medical intervention. To distinguish syncope from seizure, which also involves TLOC and spontaneous recovery, syncope is further defined as resulting from transient global cerebral hypoperfusion.

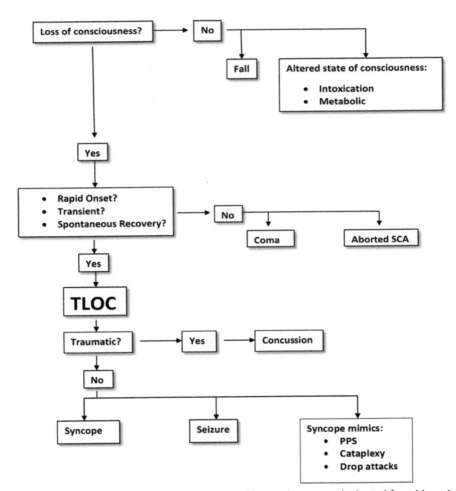

Fig. 1. Syncope in the context of TLOC. SCA, sudden cardiac arrest. (*Adapted from* Moya A, Sutton R, Ammirati F, et al. Guidelines for the diagnosis and management of syncope (version 2009). Eur Heart J 2009;21:2631–71.)

PATHOPHYSIOLOGY OF SYNCOPE

Any disturbance that results in transient self-limited inadequate cerebral perfusion may lead to syncope (**Fig. 2**).[2–4] An understanding of the pathophysiology of the syncope episode in the afflicted individual is essential to permit the clinician to evaluate the risk of recurrence, assess prognosis, and devise an appropriate treatment strategy.

Although it constitutes only approximately 2% of the body's mass, the brain receives 15% to 20% of the cardiac output at rest[5] and has little metabolic reserve. Syncope results when the brain is deprived of adequate perfusion for more than a few seconds (generally estimated as 6–10 seconds). Rossen and colleagues,[2] working in an era predating institutional review boards, occluded cerebral blood flow in 11 patients with schizophrenia and 126 normal male subjects using a pneumatic cuff placed around the lower third of the neck capable of inflating to 600 mm Hg "within one-eighth second." They found that within 5.5 seconds of flow obstruction, half the subjects developed a fixed gaze followed by slumping, indicating LOC, suggesting this time to be the maximum tolerable period of brain hypoperfusion.

In most cases, the cerebral hypoperfusion triggering syncope is the result of a brief drop of systemic perfusion pressure. In this regard, recall that systemic blood pressure (BP) is a function of both cardiac output and systemic vascular resistance. A decrease in either may result in syncope, with the pathophysiology summarized in **Fig. 3**. However, in reality, the causes of syncope are rarely so distinct. For example,

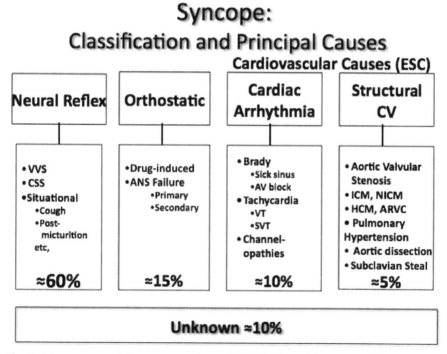

Syncope:
Classification and Principal Causes
Cardiovascular Causes (ESC)

Neural Reflex	Orthostatic	Cardiac Arrhythmia	Structural CV

• VVS
• CSS
• Situational
  • Cough
  • Post-
  micturition
  etc,
	• Drug-induced
	• ANS Failure
	  • Primary
	  • Secondary
		• Brady
		  • Sick sinus
		  • AV block
		• Tachycardia
		  • VT
		  • SVT
		• Channel-
		  opathies
			• Aortic Valvular
			  Stenosis
			• ICM, NICM
			• HCM, ARVC
			• Pulmonary
			  Hypertension
			• Aortic dissection
			• Subclavian Steal

≈60%	≈15%	≈10%	≈5%

Unknown ≈10%

Fig. 2. Scheme summarizing a commonly used classification of the causes of syncope. ANS, autonomic nervous system; ARVC, arrhythmogenic right ventricular cardiomyopathy; CSS, carotid sinus syndrome; CV, cardiovascular; ESC, European Society of Cardiology; ICM, ischemic cardiomyopathy; NICM, non-ischemic cardiomyopathy; SVT, supraventricular tachycardia; VVS, vasovagal syncope; VT, ventricular tachycardia

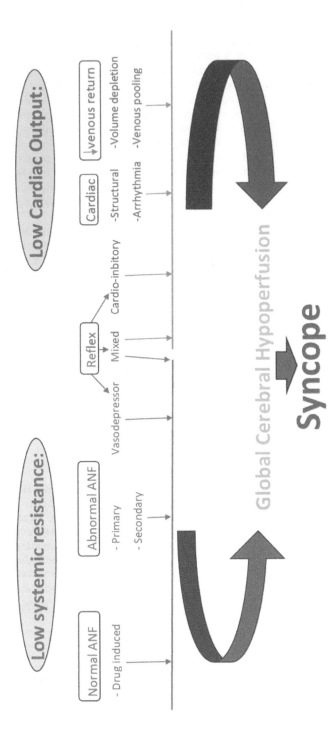

Fig. 3. Pathophysiology of syncope, any process that leads to a decrease in systemic resistance, cardiac output, or a combination may cause global cerebral hypoperfusion and syncope. ANF, Autonomic nervous system function. (*Adapted from* Moya A, Sutton R, Ammirati F, et al. Guidelines for the diagnosis and management of syncope (version 2009). Eur Heart J 2009;21:2631–71.)

cardiac syncope due to arrhythmia is most simply considered to result solely from arrhythmia-induced low cardiac output. Nevertheless, especially in the case of tachyarrhythmias, the notion that syncope results solely because the heart is "beating too fast" is overly simplistic. Careful investigations suggest that syncope in the setting of supraventricular arrhythmias may also be related to an inadequate or inappropriate vasomotor response to the arrhythmia rather than the rate of the tachycardia alone.[6,7]

The causes of syncope fall into 4 main categories, as summarized in **Fig. 2**. The large majority of patients have either one or other of the reflex syncope syndromes, also referred to as "neurallymediated," or syncope due to orthostatic hypotension (OH). This fact holds true over all age groups, including elderly individuals. For instance, among 242 individuals aged 65 to 98 years, Ungar and colleagues[8] found that the combination of neural-reflex and orthostatic faints accounted for 67% of diagnoses.

REFLEX SYNCOPE

Although not typically included under the rubric of syncope because of ANS dysfunction, reflex syncope does in fact result from the transient disturbance of autonomic regulation of cardiovascular function.

Vasovagal Syncope

Vasovagal syncope (VVS) is the most common form of reflex syncope.

If the onset of VVS is gradual, many patients (especially the younger but less often the elderly) will experience prodromal symptoms. Prodromal symptoms can result from autonomic activation or from hypoperfusion of the brain, retina, and large muscles of the neck and shoulders as well as alterations of perfusion to the splanchnic bed.[9] The presence of these prodromal symptoms is an important diagnostic clinical clue for reflex syncope. However, the absence of prodromal symptoms, especially in the elderly, does *not* exclude reflex syncope. Symptoms attributable to autonomic activation and hypoperfusion are summarized in **Box 1**.

Box 1
Prodromal symptoms in syncope

Symptoms of autonomic activation

- Sweating
- Pallor
- Nausea
- Pupillary dilation
- Hyperventilation
- Yawning
- Palpitations

Symptoms of hypoperfusion

- Brain: lightheadedness, difficulty thinking or concentrating
- Retina: tunnel vision, loss of color vision (greying out)
- Shoulders: pain across shoulders and into the neck (coat hanger pain/headache)

Adapted from Wieling W, Thijs RD, van Dijk N, et al. Symptoms and signs of syncope: a review of the link between physiology and clinical clues. Brain 2009;132:2630–42.

VVS is often viewed as the archetype of reflex syncope. Despite this, the pathophysiology of VVS remains incompletely understood. The fact that the vast majority of VVS events occur while the patient is in an upright position with the ability of a head-up tilt (HUT) table testing to trigger VVS suggests that venous pooling is a crucial element. Pooling results in a decrease in venous return to the heart, thereby diminishing cardiac output and initiating reflex increase in sympathetic tone in an attempt to maintain BP. The increase in sympathetic tone has positive chronotropic and inotropic effects. Vigorous contraction of the underfilled ventricle is thought to stimulate ventricular neural afferents to the brain; these afferents terminate in cardiovascular control centers where the visceral inputs are integrated and result in sympathetic and parasympathetic efferent neural activity to various elements of the cardiovascular system. It is thought that in VVS, activation of central nuclei leads to first accentuation, and later the abrupt withdrawal, of sympathetic tone and an increase in parasympathetic tone. The increase in parasympathetic tone tempers any attempt to provide an appropriate chronotropic response in the face of evolving hypotension resulting from sympathetic withdrawal and in many cases results in marked inappropriate heart rate (HR) slowing. Thus, both vasodepression and cardio-inhibition occur in most cases of VVS; only very rarely will a patient appear to exhibit purely "vasodepressor" or solely "cardio-inhibitory" responses based on observations during HUT testing.

The postulated explanation of VVS pathophysiology provided above is clearly incomplete. For instance, it cannot explain how emotional upset triggers VVS, or how VVS is triggered in patients after heart transplantation. In the latter, "re-innervation" is often hypothesized but that explanation is not tenable in all cases.[10–12] Furthermore, the neural pathways connecting the various vasomotor nuclei to higher cortical centers remain unknown in both VVS and situational syncope.

Carotid Sinus Syndrome and Situational Reflex Faints

Carotid sinus syndrome (CSS) is unusual in patients less than the age of 40. The "classic" history of syncope during shaving or buttoning a collar is rare. Patients may report syncope or near syncope related to movement of the head. Distinguishing near syncope due to CCS from benign positional vertigo requires careful questioning.

Situational syncope is relatively uncommon and is generally easily diagnosed by history. The most common examples are micturition syncope, cough syncope, and defecation syncope. Rarer conditions include "trumpet-blowers" syncope, swallow syncope, and the "mess-trick." In each of these cases, the "trigger" is presumably related to the specific situation; similarly, prevention is best achieved by avoiding or ameliorating the trigger situation. As in VVS, both cardio-inhibitory and vasodepressor features are usually present.

ORTHOSTATIC HYPOTENSION

As noted in **Fig. 2**, OH is the second leading cause of syncope. Drug treatment (diuretics and vasoactive agents) is the most common cause of OH and typically acts through volume depletion (eg, diuretics) or by impairing autonomic and vascular responsiveness (eg, sympatholytics, vasodilators). Primary ANS failure is relatively uncommon but its recognition is crucial for both patient education regarding prognosis and appropriate therapy.

OH may result in syncope or near syncope; in the elderly, OH is an important cause of falls and physical injury. However, many patients also exhibit a broad array of vague complaints that are better termed *orthostatic intolerance*, such as palpitations, lightheadedness, dizziness, and fatigue. The primary clinical clue is identifying that the reported symptoms are a consequence of recent movement to upright posture, or an extended period of either standing or less often a prolonged period of sitting with the legs in a dependent position.

A 2011 consensus statement refined the definition of OH and incorporated several common variants (**Table 1**).[13] Gibbons and Freeman[14] reported that in 230 patients undergoing HUT testing 46% developed OH in less than 3 minutes, 15% between 3 and 10 minutes, and in 39% of the patients OH was not seen until greater than 10 minutes of HUT. Adding to the diagnostic complexity, there are patients who have delayed OH in conjunction with reflex syncope and those in whom reflex syncope is triggered by assuming an upright posture. HUT testing may be helpful to distinguish these cases from classical or delayed OH.

Primary Autonomic Nervous System Failure

Primary disorders of ANS function are rare or infrequent causes of OH. Several are associated with precipitation of α-synuclein in either glial cells, cytoplasm of populations, or neurons or both and have been referred to as the synucleinopathies.[15] Patients with primary ANS failure often have supine hypertension, which can complicate treatment of OH.

Parkinson disease

Patients with Parkinson disease not infrequently develop OH. In Parkinson disease, autonomic dysfunction appears relatively late.[15,16] The degree of autonomic dysfunction is typically less than in multisystem atrophy (MSA). OH may also be exacerbated by certain anti-Parkinsonism medications, particularly levodopa and bromocriptine (**Box 2**).

Multiple-system atrophy also known as Shy-Drager syndrome

Severe autonomic dysfunction develops early and in some patients may be the most prominent clinical feature.[15,17] Other features include Parkinsonism, dysarthria, dystonia and contractures, rapid eye movement sleep disorders, and dementia.

Table 1
Classification of orthostatic hypotension

Classification	Diagnostic Test	Time to Onset of Symptoms
Initial OH	• Active standing • With beat-to-beat BP measurement	0–30 s
Classical OH	• Active standing • HUT testing	30 s to 3 min
Delayed OH	• HUT tilt • Active standing >3 min • Progressive decrease in BP without bradycardia • In ANF may not see appropriate reflex tachycardia	3–30 min
Delayed OH plus Reflex syncope	• HUT with progressive decrease in BP, then abrupt decrease in HR and BP typical of VVS	3–30 min
VVS triggered by standing	• HUT with normal initial response to standing followed by abrupt drop in HR and BP	3–30 min

Adapted from Freeman R, Wieling W, Axelord FB, et al. Consensus statement on the definition of orthostatic hypotension, neutrally mediated syncope and the postural tachycardia syndrome. Auton Neurosci 2011;161:46–8.

Box 2
Drugs that commonly cause orthostatic hypotension

- Diuretics
- α-Adrenergic receptor antagonists
  - Prazosin
  - Doxazosin
  - Terazosin
- β-Adrenergic receptor blockers
- Combined α- and β-adrenergic receptor blockers
  - Labetalol
  - Carvedilol
- Anti-Parkinson medications
  - Bromocriptine
  - Levodopa
  - Pramipexole
- Tricyclic antidepressants
- Phosphodiesterase type 5 inhibitors
- Atypical antipsychotics
  - Lurasidone
  - Risperadone
  - Sertindole
- Monoamine oxidase inhibitors

Lewy-body dementia

Autonomic dysfunction occurs early.[15,18] Dementia may precede or coincide with Parkinsonism. Lewy-bodies are precipitates of α-synuclein within the cytoplasm of central nervous system neurons.

Pure autonomic failure

Patients with pure autonomic failure (PAF) do not have motor symptoms and only rarely progress to Parkinson disease or Lewy-body dementia.[15,19] Clinically, they often present with symptoms of OH or orthostatic intolerance related to exercise or immediately after exercise. They generally respond well to therapy and their prognosis is generally better than in the other primary autonomic disorders.

Secondary Autonomic Nervous System Failure

The most frequent cause of OH is medications; the most important of these medications are listed in **Box 2**.

Excluding medications, diabetes is the next most frequent cause of ANS dysfunction in the developed world. Diabetics with OH often, but not always, have polyneuropathy with associated gastroparesis, diarrhea, constipation, urinary retention, and erectile dysfunction. On occasion, OH occurs early in the course of the disease.[20]

Primary amyloidosis (light-chain amyloidosis) and hereditary amyloidosis also cause secondary autonomic dysfunction that frequently results in OH.[21] Gingival or rectal biopsies or examination of fat aspirates will reveal the presence of amyloid.

Hereditary amyloidosis presents earlier in life and is most commonly related to mutant form of transthyretin. Genetic testing or immunohistochemical staining is needed to distinguish between primary and hereditary amyloidosis. There are 2 clues on physical examination. Macroglossia and periorbital purpura are seen in primary amyloidosis but not in the hereditary form. Both conditions are associated with a polyneuropathy. Primary amyloidosis progresses more rapidly than hereditary amyloidosis.[22]

Postural tachycardia syndrome (POTS) is often included in discussions of OH, although it is better considered as orthostatic intolerance because hypotension is unusual in POTS. It is characterized by a symptomatic increase in the HR on standing. However, *by definition,* the increase in HR is NOT associated with OH and usually not associated with syncope. POTS is a poorly understood condition that often afflicts a younger group of patients than is usually bothered by OH and will not be discussed further in this review.

CARDIAC SYNCOPE

Approximately 15% of syncope is of a cardiac cause (see **Fig. 2**), either arrhythmic or related to structural cardiac disease. As already noted,[6,7] ANS dysfunction may play a role in cardiac syncope secondary to tachyarrhythmia; this is also true for atrial fibrillation,[23] sinus bradycardia,[24] pulmonary embolus,[25] aortic stenosis,[26,27] and hypertrophic cardiomyopathy.[28]

Syncope in the setting of myocardial infarction may be related to ischemia or infarction of specialized conduction system tissue. Reflex-mediated syncope in the setting of inferior and inferoposterior infarction (ie, the Bezold-Jarish reflex or more correctly von Bezold-Jarish) is often encountered clinically.[29]

Reflex-mediated mechanisms may play a role in ventricular tachyarrhythmias as well. Rare but potentially lethal disorders, such as the long QT syndromes, short QT syndrome, and Brugada syndrome, can be diagnosed from a standard 12-lead electrocardiogram (ECG).

Mortality is a greater concern in cardiac syncope than among individuals with syncope and no structural disease; early and accurate diagnosis of cardiac syncope is critical.[30] Clinical features suggesting high risk are summarized in **Box 3**.

EVALUATION OF THE PATIENT WITH SYNCOPE

The goal of the evaluation is to establish a specific cause for the patient's syncope to facilitate a discussion of the treatment options and likely future course of the disease. However, first one must be certain that the patient has in fact suffered a syncopal episode.

As noted in the introduction and as diagrammed in **Fig. 1**, LOC is an obligatory part of the definition of syncope, and if it has not occurred, the patient, by definition, did not have syncope. LOC inevitably leads to loss of postural tone, and unless restrained, the affected patient will, voluntarily or otherwise, seek a gravitationally neutral position; they will fall or slump over. A report of LOC in an unrestrained patient who did not fall or slump, or who remains down for many minutes, raises the possibility of psychogenic pseudosyncope (PPS), which will be discussed later.

Differentiating syncope from a seizure can be difficult. Eyewitnesses will often report jerking movements in patients with syncope. A detailed history is critical, and neurologic consultation may be needed, in making the distinction.[31,32] A careful comprehensive history is far more helpful than brain imaging or the routine use of electroencephalograms (EEGs) in the absence of head trauma or a high index of suspicion for a seizure disorder based on the history (**Table 2**).

Box 3
Risk stratification: high-risk features suggesting the need for hospitalization

Structural heart disease

- Low ejection fraction
- Prior myocardial infarction
- Heart failure
- Implantable cardioverter defibrillator or permanent pacemaker present

Clinical findings

- Syncope during active exercise
- Syncope while supine
- Palpitations before syncope
- Family history of sudden cardiac death, familial cardiomyopathy, or channelopathy

Electrocardiographic findings

- Nonsustained ventricular tachycardia
- Bifascicular block
- Nonspecific intraventricular conduction delay with QRS greater than 120 ms
- Ventricular pre-excitation
- Second-degree heart block, type II
- Sinus bradycardia, HR less than 50 bpm while awake and in absence of negative chronotropic drugs or physical conditioning
- Long or short QT interval
- Brugada pattern: right bundle branch block with ST elevation in V1–V3[a]
- Negative T wave in V1–V2 (in adults) with εwave[a]

[a] ECG examples can be found at: http://en.ecgpedia.org/wiki/Main_Page.
Adapted from Moya A, Sutton R, Ammirati F, et al. Guidelines for the diagnosis and management of syncope (version 2009). Eur Heart J 2009;21:2631–71.

True syncope is transient, rarely lasting longer than a minute. Patients with very frequent episodes, sometimes daily, or apparent LOC that is prolonged, often lasting several minutes, are more likely to be suffering from PPS. In these patients, ambulatory ECG monitoring can be helpful in documenting that the symptoms are not related to an arrhythmia (although vasodepressor faints cannot be absolutely excluded). HUT testing is also useful in that PPS can often be induced with tilt testing. The apparent LOC will not be associated with a drop in HR or BP. EEG and video monitoring during tilt offer additional evidence that the apparent LOC does not have a demonstrable hypotensive or arrhythmic physiologic basis.[33,34]

Cataplexy and drop attacks are relatively rare disorders that mimic syncope. The critical distinction is that these disorders do not result in LOC. Cataplexy is often associated with narcolepsy. It is characterized by the abrupt loss of muscle tone triggered by emotion, often laughter.[35,36]

The term "drop attack" has been used, or misused, to describe a variety of events. It is has become commonly used as a synonym for a Stokes-Adams attack (ie, an abrupt LOC spell most often due to transient atrioventricular block). In its original sense, it describes the sudden loss of motor control, almost exclusively in middle-aged women,

Table 2
Clinical features: syncope versus epilepsy

Favors Seizure	Favors Syncope
Before the event	
Blue face	Diaphoresis, nausea, abdominal pain, lightheadedness
Aura	Visual disturbances: tunnel vision, shooting stars
	Auditory disturbances: roaring, muffled
Eyewitness observations during the event	
Tonic-clonic movements coincide with LOC	Jerky movements after LOC
Movements of relatively long duration	Brief duration
Automatisms such as lip smacking, chewing	
Involvement of only one side or lateralizing movements	
After the event	
Tongue biting, especially sides of tongue	Fatigue of variable duration
Prolonged confusion	Confusion, if present, is brief
Muscle aches	
Findings that are NOT helpful in distinguishing seizure from syncope	
Urinary incontinence	
Injury (other than tongue biting)	
Family history of seizure	
Headache	
Drowsiness	

Adapted from Moya A, Sutton R, Ammirati F, et al. Guidelines for the diagnosis and management of syncope (version 2009). Eur Heart J 2009;21:2631–71.

who typically fell to their knees. Furthermore, in a "drop attack," the patient does not suffer LOC and maintains awareness and recall of the event. An additional complexity, however, is that many patients may not recollect having had LOC; consequently, true syncope (especially due to delayed OH) may be overlooked on initial evaluation.

ESTABLISHING THE CAUSE OF THE SYNCOPE

The initial assessment of the patient with syncope is focused on making a diagnosis and establishing the patient's risk for future events or death. A comprehensive medical history is of paramount importance. In many cases, the experienced clinician will have a probable diagnosis after taking the history. In most cases, the physical examination and any further testing should be selected carefully to confirm the suspected diagnosis. Undirected screening diagnostic testing strategies are expensive and rarely fruitful.

Pooled data from population-based studies indicate that the history and physical examination identify a potential cause of syncope in approximately 50% of the patients.[8,37–42] Reflex syncope (vasovagal, situational) accounts for approximately 75% of diagnoses at initial evaluation. The diagnostic yield of standard ECG obtained in the emergency department is on average 6% and accounts for about the half of total diagnoses of cardiac syncope. In-hospital (telemetry) monitoring is helpful in a minority of selected high-risk patients.[38]

CRITICAL FEATURES OF THE HISTORY

The history should include all aspects of the event, including circumstances before the event, prodromal symptoms, eyewitness description of the event itself (when available), associated injuries, and recovery from the event. The patients should be questioned about known cardiac disease, medications (in particular, new medications or recent dose changes), prior syncope, and diseases, such as diabetes or Parkinson disease, that are often associated with ANS failure.[1]

If the initial assessment suggests that syncope was due to OH, a more detailed history focusing on evidence of other manifestations of autonomic dysfunction is warranted. Findings that raise suspicion of OH and ANS failure include the following:

- Syncope after standing
- Syncope during or shortly after exercise
- Diabetes, especially in patients with other symptoms of generalized diabetic neuropathy
- Long-standing Parkinson disease
- Elderly, especially those in long-term care facilities

Clinical features that suggest autonomic system failure are summarized in **Box 4**. For a more detailed review of the medical history in the evaluation of syncope, the interested reader may refer to the 2009 article by Wieling and colleagues.[9]

PHYSICAL EXAMINATION

The initial examination should include a complete physical examination, orthostatic vital signs, and an ECG. Orthostatic vital signs should be measured starting with the patient having rested in a supine position for a few minutes. After the supine baseline measurements are completed, the patient should stand (so-called active standing test). The BP and HR are remeasured 30 to 60 seconds after standing and every 1 to 2 minutes thereafter for a minimum of 5 minutes.

The physical examination is focused on identifying patients with structural heart disease and is often assisted by echocardiographic imaging. The routine examination should include an assessment of gait and stability. If the history suggests autonomic dysfunction, a neurology consultation is recommended.

The 12-lead ECG is an important part of the initial evaluation of patients with TLOC and suspected syncope. The ECG may suggest underlying structural heart disease such as left ventricular hypertrophy, right ventricular strain, conduction system disease, or prior myocardial infarction. Similarly, the ECG may identify ion channel mutations (so-called channelopathies) such as occur in long QT syndrome or Brugada syndrome; these are rare but potentially life-threatening causes of syncope. Overall, ECG findings do not often provide proof positive evidence of a basis for syncope, but an abnormal finding offers direction for further assessment.

In patients more than age 40 or 50, or having a history of syncope related to movements of the head or neck, carotid sinus massage (CSM) should be performed by an individual experienced with this procedure. CSM should be done during continuous ECG and BP monitoring (the latter preferably using beat-to-beat recordings because otherwise a prominent vasodepressor response may be missed). In addition, CSM can be most effectively used if the patient is in an upright posture, such as on a tilt-table. CSM is considered diagnostic if it reproduces syncope symptoms associated with greater than 3 seconds of asystole or a drop in SBP greater than 50 mm Hg.[1]

Box 4
Important findings in the autonomic history

OH or intolerance

- Lightheadedness/dizziness

- Weakness

- Neck and shoulder pain, "coat hanger" headache thought to be due to ischemia of the neck and shoulder muscles secondary to hypotension

- Visual changes: "tunnel vision" less common than blurring, inability to focus, on occasion visual hallucination suggests occipital lobe ischemia

- Worsening of symptoms of intolerance by

  ○ Eating

  ○ Alcohol

  ○ Early morning

  ○ Hot shower, bath, or hot environment

  ○ Exercise

  ○ Bed rest

Cutaneous

- Abnormal sweating: hypohidrosis in some areas with hyperhidrosis in others

Gastrointestinal

- Early satiety, postprandial fullness

- Constipation

- Diarrhea

- Fecal urgency

Genitourinary

- Urinary frequency/retention

- Erectile dysfunction

- Abnormal ejaculation

Adapted from Robertson D. Clinical assessment of autonomic failure. In: Robertson D, editor. Primer on the autonomic nervous system. Amsterdam: Elsevier Academic Press; 2004. p. 213–6.

Routine blood tests rarely yield diagnostically useful information. In selected syncope cases, they can confirm a clinical suspicion of acute anemia, myocardial infarction, or pulmonary embolism. Very rarely, such tests may yield other nonsyncope TLOC diagnoses, such as hypoglycemia and intoxications.

ANCILLARY TESTING

Ancillary testing should be limited to studies needed to confirm a diagnosis. In particular, echocardiography is an invaluable tool for establishing the presence or absence of structural heart disease. An echocardiogram should be obtained if either the history or the physical examination suggests structural heart disease.[1]

Tilt Table Testing

Tilt table testing is most effectively used in patients with suspected VVS but atypical histories, or patients with evidence of structural heart disease but with a presentation suggesting VVS as the cause of syncope. In these latter cases, the goal is to confirm a suspected VVS diagnosis. Tilt-table testing can help to distinguish OH from VVS or to identify patients who may have a combination of OH and VVS. The 2009 European Society of Cardiology guidelines provide recommendations regarding tilt-testing methodology, indications, and diagnostic criteria.[1]

Ambulatory Electrocardiographic Monitoring

Electrocardiographic monitoring, especially by means of implantable loop recorders, is extremely helpful in establishing an arrhythmic cause for syncope. They are of limited use in patients with ANS failure where the primary cause of syncope is OH.

Exercise Testing

Exercise testing is indicated when syncope occurs during exercise or shortly after exercise. Syncope occurring during exercise is considered a high-risk presentation. When exercise results in hypotension, it suggests either structural heart disease extensive enough to prevent an adequate increase in cardiac output, the inability to regulate blood flow to nonworking vascular beds, or exercise-induced arrhythmias.

Electrophysiology Study

Electrophysiology study (EPS) has little value in helping to define syncope because of autonomic disturbances related to either transient ANS dysfunction or ANS failure and will not be discussed further.

Computed Tomography, MRI, Electroencephalogram, Carotid Ultrasound

In patients with no trauma to the head and a nonfocal neurologic examination, there is no indication for brain imaging; this is especially the case if an autonomic basis for syncope- is deemed likely.

AUTONOMIC NERVOUS SYSTEM TESTING

ANS testing can be helpful in identifying patients with fixed or progressive ANS failure as opposed to those with transient ANS dysfunction seen in VVS and other reflex syncope syndromes.

VALSALVA MANEUVER

Performance of the Valsalva maneuver allows for evaluation of baroreceptor, sympathetic, and parasympathetic function.[43] The maneuver is performed by having the patient blow into a mouthpiece connected to an aneroid BP gauge. The mouthpiece should have a small air leak to avoid closure of the glottis. The patient is instructed to maintain a pressure of 40 mm Hg for 15 to 20 seconds while beat-to-beat HR and BP measurements are recorded. The normal HR and BP response to the Valsalva maneuver is divided into 4 phases, as summarized in **Box 5**.

A commonly used measure is the Valsalva ratio. The Valsalva ratio is the ratio of the shortest RR (tachycardia) interval after phase 2 to the longest RR interval (bradycardia) in phase 4. Age- and gender-based norms have been established for the Valsalva ratio.[44]

Box 5
Phases of the Valsalva maneuver

Phase 1

- Increase in intrathoracic pressure leads to compression of the aorta and propulsion of blood into the circulation leading to a transient increase in BP. This increase in BP is due to mechanical effects and is not dependent on sympathetic activation.
- Arteriolar baroreceptors and pulmonary stretch receptors are activated leading to a decrease in BP and HR in late phase 1 and the early portion of phase 2.

Phase 2

- In the early phase, BP and cardiac output continue to decrease because of marked impairment in venous return.
- The decrease in cardiac output results in reflex sympathetic activation via the arterial baroreceptors.
- Reflex sympathetic activation results in recovery of BP late in phase 2.

Phase 3

- Expiration ends resulting in a drop in intrathoracic pressure leading to a mechanical drop in BP.

Phase 4

- Venous return to the heart increases and cardiac output increases.
- Systemic resistance remains high.
- Increased cardiac output in the face of increased systemic resistance results in an increase in BP above baseline, the "overshoot."
- Baroreceptor activation results in slowing of the HR.

Adapted from Looga R. The Valsalva manoeuvre—cardiovascular effects and performance technique: a critical review. Resp Physiol Neurobiol. 2005;147:39–49; with permission.

Tests of Sympathetic Adrenergic Function

Sympathetic function is frequently tested with very little awareness on the part of the clinician that that is what is being done; specifically, the BP response to postural changes such as active standing or HUT. Failure to maintain BP in the face of postural stress represents a failure of sympathetic vascular control function. The increase in HR on assuming an upright posture is due to both withdrawal of vagal tone and an increase in sympathetic tone. Failure of the HR to increase in response to a continued decrease in BP also reflects sympathetic dysfunction.

The BP response to the Valsalva maneuver provides insights regarding sympathetic function. Recovery of BP in late phase 2 and the overshoot in BP seen in phase 4 are mediated by increases in sympathetic tone. Failure of the BP to recover in phase 2 or to overshoot in phase 4 are markers of failure to increase sympathetic tone.

Testing of sudomotor function is available in a few specialized centers.[45] Common tests for sudomotor function include the following:

- Quantitative sudomotor axon reflex test
- Thermoregulatory sweat test
- Skin imprint and skin potential recordings

All of these methods are time-consuming and most require specialized equipment, limiting their clinical utility.

TREATMENT OF SPECIFIC CONDITIONS
Reflex Syncope

There are no large well-controlled trials demonstrating efficacy of the commonly used approaches to the treatment of VVS. The mainstay of therapy remains education on the avoidance of triggers and adequate salt and fluid intake. The current controversy regarding salt restrictions is not touched upon here, except to note that many of the patients seen have a near phobia when it comes to increasing their salt intake. In selected patients, pharmacologic agents may be used.[1] Situational syncope is treated by avoiding or ameliorating the situation that results in syncope. CSS is the one reflex syncope that is commonly and generally very effectively treated with cardiac pacing.[1]

Orthostatic Hypotension and Intolerance

Medication-related OH is best managed by reducing the dosage or discontinuing the drug when possible. Patients and clinicians may find they must accept BP higher than typically accepted as ideal to avoid debilitating orthostatic syncope or intolerance.

The importance of adequate salt and fluid intake cannot be overemphasized. Patients are instructed to measure their salt intake and at times may require up to 10 g of sodium daily. Fluid intake should be at least 2.0 to 2.5 L daily. A 24-hour urine test can be useful in documenting adequate sodium and fluid intake. The urinary sodium should be greater than 170 mmol and urine volume greater than 1500 mL/24 hours.[46]

Other lifestyle interventions include the following:

- Gradual, staged changes in postural position
- To minimize postprandial OH, frequent small meals, avoidance of alcohol with meals, and a minimum of 8 ounces of water with the meal
- To minimize morning symptoms, 12 to 20 ounces of water, taken rapidly 10 to 15 minutes before getting out of bed and delaying shower or bath until after adequate hydration
- Elevate the head of the bed 6 to 10 inches to reduce supine hypertension and nocturnal diuresis
- Avoid prolonged recumbency/bed rest
- Continue isotonic exercises, recumbent exercise may be more easily tolerated
- Abdominal binders (20 mm Hg pressure) and waist-high compression garments may be of benefit. Patients may find Lycra bike shorts, with both abdominal and thigh compression, to be more comfortable and efficacious.

In patients who remain symptomatic despite lifestyle modifications, pharmacologic therapy may be required. Until recently, midodrine was the only drug approved by the US Food and Drug Administration (FDA) for the treatment of OH. Midodrine is a direct α1-adrenergic receptor agonist. The dose varies from 2.5 to 10.0 mg. It has a short half-life and can be taken every 4 to 6 hours. Patients should not take midodrine within 4 hours of returning to a recumbent position because of the potential to exacerbate supine hypertension. Midodrine may cause urinary retention, especially in elderly men. In patients with OH who are taking an α-adrenergic agonist for urinary retention, the best course would be to stop the α-adrenergic agonist, if possible. Midodrine may also cause pilomotor reactions and pruritis.

Droxidopa is a prodrug that undergoes decarboxylation to norepinephrine by L-aromatic amino acid decarboxylase. In both European and US trials, it was found to be a safe and effective treatment for OH due to Parkinson disease, MSA, and PAF.[47,48] Droxidopa has been approved by the FDA for the treatment of neurogenic OH.

Fluodrocortisone is often used for volume expansion. Frequently, patients with OH also have supine hypertension, which may be increased with the use of fluodrocortisone. Patients receiving fluodrocortisone should have their potassium levels monitored regularly because this medication may cause hypokalemia. Regularly monitored potassium levels is especially important if the patient is taking digoxin or an antiarrhythmic drug. In the authors' practice, midodrine, with its short duration of action, is preferred when tolerated.

It is important to educate the patient to expect an increase in ankle edema associated with increased sodium intake or with the use of fluodrocortisone. It is not uncommon for patients, who had been doing well on therapy, to return to clinic because of a worsening of their symptoms after having resumed diuretic therapy for edema.

Supine hypertension can be a major complicating factor in the treatment of OH. Raising the head of the bed 6 to 10 inches reduces supine hypertension. When treatment of supine hypertension is needed, the authors prefer to use a short-acting agent, such as captopril, given at bedtime. A great deal of time is required to educate the patient on how they may adjust their medications (antihypertensives and midodrine) based on their BP readings and anticipated activities. In addition, they should be warned about OH recurrence if getting up in the night to go to the bathroom. A bedside commode or walker may be helpful to prevent falls at night.

Other medications that have been used to treat OH related to autonomic dysfunction include intranasal desmopression[49] and erythropoietin.[50] These medications are infrequently used. With the FDA approval of droxidopa, the use of these agents for OH is likely to continue to decline.

SUMMARY

Syncope is a common problem seen in all clinical practices. It can result from any number of disorders that lead to inadequate perfusion of the brain. A thorough and focused history is essential to arriving at the correct diagnosis. In many cases, a diagnosis can be reached without the need for additional testing. Syncope due to reflex syncope (i.e., transient ANS dysfunction such as in the vasovagal faint) is by far the most common. Patients with rare episodes of reflex syncope (excluding CSS) require no additional testing and no therapy beyond education and lifestyle modification. Syncope due to fixed or progressive ANS dysfunction is rare but is easily overlooked, often being dismissed as a simple fact of aging. OH due to fixed ANS dysfunction adds a significant burden to a patient already struggling with a neurologic disorder such as Parkinson or MSA (multisystem atrophy). Accurate diagnosis is essential if the clinician is to effectively educate the patient regarding prognosis and initiate appropriate therapy.

REFERENCES

1. Moya A, Sutton R, Ammirati F, et al. Guidelines for the diagnosis and management of syncope (version 2009). Eur Heart J 2009;21:2631–71.
2. Rossen R, Kabat H, Anderson JP. Acute arrest of cerebral circulation in man. Arch Neurol Psychiatry 1943;50:510–28.
3. Blanc JJ, Benditt DG. Syncope: definition, classification, and multiple potential causes. In: Benditt DG, Blanc JJ, Brignole M, et al, editors. The evaluation and treatment of syncope. A handbook for clinical practice. Elmsford (NY): Futura Blackwell; 2003. p. 3–10.
4. van Dijk JG, Thijs RD, Benditt DG, Wieling W. A guide to disorders causing transient loss of consciousness: focus on syncope. Nat Rev Neurol 2009;5:438–48.

5. van Lieshout JJ, Wieling W, Karemaker JM, et al. Syncope, cerebral perfusion, and oxygenation. J Appl Physiol 2003;94:833–48.
6. Leitch JW, Klein GJ, Yee R, et al. Syncope associated with supraventricular tachycardia: an expression of tachycardia or vasomotor response? Circulation 1992;85:1064–71.
7. Doi A, Miyamoto K, Uno K, et al. Studies on hemodynamic instability in paroxysmal supraventricular tachycardia: noninvasive evaluations by head-up tilt testing and power spectrum analysis on electrocardiographic RR variation. Pacing Clin Electrophysiol 2003;23:1623–31.
8. Ungar A, Mussi C, Del Rosso A, et al. Study of syncope for the italian group for the study of syncope in the elderly. Diagnosis and characteristics of syncope in older patients referred to geriatric departments. J Am Geriatr Soc 2006;54:1531–6.
9. Wieling W, Thijs RD, van Dijk N, et al. Symptoms and signs of syncope: a review of the link between physiology and clinical clues. Brain 2009;132:2630–42.
10. Fitzpatrick AP, Banner N, Cheng A, et al. Vasovagal reactions may occur after orthotopic heart transplantation. J Am Coll Cardiol 1993;21:1132–7.
11. Morgan-Hughes NJ, Dark JH, McComb JM, et al. Vasovagal reactions after heart transplantation. J Am Coll Cardiol 1993;22(7):2059.
12. Montebugnoli L, Montanari G. Vasovagal syncope in heart transplant patients during dental surgery. Oral Surg Oral Med Oral Pathol Oral Radiol Endod 1999;87(6):666–9.
13. Freeman R, Wieling W, Axelord FB, et al. Consensus statement of the definition of orthostatic hypotension, neutrally mediated syncope and the postural tachycardia syndrome. Auton Neurosci 2011;161:46–8.
14. Gibbons CH, Freeman R. Delayed orthostatic hypotension: a frequent cause of orthostatic intolerance. Neurology 2006;67:28–32.
15. Freeman R. Neurogenic orthostatic hypotension. N Engl J Med 2008;358:615–24.
16. Davis TL. Parkinson's disease. In: Robertson D, editor. Primer on the autonomic nervous system. Amsterdam: Elsevier Academic Press; 2004. p. 287–9.
17. Quinn N. Multiple system atrophy. In: Robertson D, editor. Primer on the autonomic nervous system. Amsterdam: Elsevier Academic Press; 2004. p. 290–2.
18. Wenning GK, Stampfer M. Dementia with Lewy bodies. In: Robertson D, editor. Primer on the autonomic nervous system. Amsterdam: Elsevier Academic Press; 2004. p. 287–9.
19. Kaufmann H, Schatz IJ. Pure autonomic. In: Robertson D, editor. Primer on the autonomic nervous system. Amsterdam: Elsevier Academic Press; 2004. p. 287–9.
20. Low PA, Benrud-Larson LM, Sletten DM, et al. Autonomic symptoms and diabetic neuropathy: a population-based study. Diabetes 2004;27:2942–7.
21. Adams D. Hereditary and acquired amyloid neuropathies. J Neurol 2001;248:647–57.
22. Ruberg FL, Berk JL. Transthyretin (TTR) cardiac amyloidosis. Circulation 2012;126:1286–300.
23. Brignole M, Gianfranchi L, Menozzi C, et al. Role of autonomic reflexes in syncope associated with paroxysmal atrial fibrillation. J Am Coll Cardiol 1993;22:1123–9.
24. Alboni P, Menozzi C, Brignole M, et al. An abnormal neural reflex plays a role in causing syncope in sinus bradycardia. J Am Coll Cardiol 1993;22:1130–4.
25. Eldadah ZA, Najjar SS, Ziegelstein RC. A patient with syncope, only "vagally" related to the heart. Chest 2000;11:1801–3.

26. Grech ED, Ramsdale DR. Exertional syncope in aortic stenosis: evidence to support inappropriate left ventricular baroreceptor response. Am Heart J 1991;121:603–6.
27. Richards AM, Nicholls MG, Ikram H, et al. Syncope in aortic valvular stenosis. Lancet 1984;2:1113–6.
28. Thomson HL, Morris-Thurgood J, Atherton J, et al. Reduced cardiopulmonary baroreflex sensitivity in patients with hypertrophic cardiomyopathy. J Am Coll Cardiol 1998;31:1377–82.
29. Mark AL. The Bezold-Jarisch reflex revisited: clinical implications of inhibitory reflexes originating in the heart. J Am Coll Cardiol 1983;1:90–102.
30. Kapoor WN, Karpf M, Wieand S, et al. A prospective evaluation and follow-up of patients with syncope. N Engl J Med 1983;309:197–204.
31. Hoefnagels WA, Padberg GW, Overweg J, et al. Transient loss of consciousness: the value of the history for distinguishing seizure from syncope. J Neurol 1991; 238:39–43.
32. Sheldon R, Rose S, Ritchie D, et al. Historical criteria that distinguish syncope from seizures. J Am Coll Cardiol 2002;40:142–8.
33. Tannemaat MR, van Niekerk J, Reijntjes RH, et al. The semiology of tilt-induced psychogenic pseudosyncope. Neurology 2013;81:752–8.
34. van Dijk JG, Wieling W. Pathophysiological basis of syncope and neurological conditions that mimic syncope. Prog Cardiovasc Dis 2013;55:345–56.
35. Lammers GJ, Overeem S, Tijssen MA, et al. Effects of startle and laughter in cataplectic subjects: a neurophysiological study between attacks. Clin Neurophysiol 2000;111:1276–81.
36. Burgess CR, Scammell TE. Narcolepsy: neural mechanisms of sleepiness and cataplexy. J Neurosci 2012;32:12305–11.
37. Del Ross A, Ungar A, Maggi R, et al. Clinical predictors of cardiac syncope at initial evaluation in patients referred urgently to a general hospital: the EGSYS score. Heart 2008;94:1620–6.
38. Benezet-Mazuecos J, Ibanez G, Rubio JM, et al. Utility of in-hospital cardiac remote telemetry in patients with unexplained syncope. Europace 2007;9: 1196–201.
39. Brignole M, Ungar A, Casagranda I, et al. Prospective multicentre systematic guideline-based management of patients referred to the Syncope Units of general hospitals. Europace 2010;12:109–18.
40. Serletis A, Rose S, Sheldon AG, et al. Vasovagal syncope in medical students and their first-degree relatives. Eur Heart J 2006;27:1965–70.
41. Sumner GL, Rose MS, Koshman ML, et al. Prevention of syncope trial investigators. Recent history of vasovagal syncope in a young, referral-based population is a stronger predictor of recurrent syncope than lifetime syncope burden. J Cardiovasc Electrophysiol 2010;21:1375–80.
42. Brignole M, Menozzi C, Bartoletti A, et al. A new management of syncope: prospective systematic guideline-based evaluation of patients referred urgently to general hospitals. Eur Heart J 2006;27:76–82.
43. Looga R. The Valsalva manoeuvre—cardiovascular effects and performance technique: a critical review. Resp Physiol Neurobiol 2005;147:39–49.
44. Low PA, Denq JC, Opfer-Gehrking TL, et al. Effect of age and gender on sudomotor and cardiovagal function and blood pressure response to tilt in normal subjects. Muscle Nerve 1997;20:1561–8.
45. Low PA, Schondorf R. Assessment of sudomotor function. In: Robertson D, editor. Primer on the autonomic nervous system. Amsterdam: Elsevier Academic Press; 2004. p. 231–3.

46. Wieling W, van Lieshout JJ, Hainsworth R. Extracellular fluid volume expansion in patients with posturally related syncope. Clin Auton Res 2002;12:242–9.
47. Kaufmann H. L-dihydroxyphenylserine (Droxidopa): a new therapy for neurogenic orthostatic hypotension: the US experience. Clin Auton Res 2008; 18(Suppl 1):19–24.
48. Mathias CJ. L-dihydroxyphenylserine (Droxidopa) in the treatment of orthostatic hypotension: the European experience. Clin Auton Res 2008;18(Suppl 1):25–9.
49. Sakakibara R, Matsuda S, Uchiyama T, et al. The effect of intranasal desmopressin on nocturnal waking in urination in multiple system atrophy patients with nocturnal polyuria. Clin Auton Res 2003;13:106–8.
50. Perera R, Isola L, Kaufmann H. Effect of recombinant erythropoietin on anemia and orthostatic hypertension in primary autonomic failure. Clin Auton Res 1995; 5:211–3.

Cardiovascular Disease Risk Assessment and Prevention

Current Guidelines and Limitations

Peter Alagona Jr, MD[a],*, Tariq Ali Ahmad, MD[b]

KEYWORDS

- Atherosclerotic cardiovascular disease • Cardiovascular disease
- Peripheral arterial disease • Risk assessment • Clinical guideline(s)

KEY POINTS

- Even with decades of progress in understanding atherosclerotic cardiovascular disease (ASCVD) and improved cardiovascular (CV) event prevention, the incidence, consequences, and cost of cardiovascular disease remain a significant public health issue.
- Observational studies have identified major ASCVD risk factors; however, a significant number of those at risk are not identified and most recurrent CV events still take place after aggressive prevention strategies are used.
- The statin era helped revolutionize clinical practice not only by effective outcome-driven low-density lipoprotein-cholesterol reduction but also by encouraging across-the-board aggressive prevention efforts.
- There are now numerous clinical guidelines for ASCVD risk stratification and treatment recommendations promulgated over the last 3 decades.
- Few patients are alike, and providing patient-centered care using all the tools available including, but not exclusively, evidence and clinical recommendations is paramount.

INTRODUCTION

Atherosclerotic cardiovascular disease (ASCVD) affects more than one-third of the adult population, accounts for 35% of all US deaths, and is a leading cause of disability. ASCVD kills more women each year than the next 3 causes of death combined. More than 50% of ASCVD presents as coronary events, including sudden cardiac death, nonfatal myocardial infarction (MI), and revascularization, with the rest being stroke and claudication associated with peripheral arterial disease.[1] The last

[a] Penn State Heart and Vascular Institute, Penn State Milton S. Hershey Medical Center, University Drive, Rm C5833, P.O.Box 850, Hershey, PA 17033-0850, USA; [b] Division of General Internal Medicine, Penn State Milton S. Hershey Medical Center, 500 University Drive, Hershey, PA 17033, USA
* Corresponding author.
E-mail address: palagona@hmc.psu.edu

Med Clin N Am 99 (2015) 711–731
http://dx.doi.org/10.1016/j.mcna.2015.02.003
0025-7125/15/$ – see front matter © 2015 Elsevier Inc. All rights reserved.

medical.theclinics.com

4 decades have witnessed unrelenting advances in the understanding of atherogenesis and development of clinically manifest ASCVD, including epidemiology, natural history, pathophysiology, risk assessment of, and treatments. Hallmarks of this disease process include:

- Begins decades before clinical manifestations,[2,3]
- Can involve a variety of different vascular beds with myriad presentations,
- Can be to a substantial degree prevented or modified.[4]

The atherosclerotic process is complex and appears to be initiated by the entrance and retention of atherogenic apolipoprotein B (apoB) particles (**Box 1**)[5] in the arterial subendothelial space. However, as noted in **Fig. 1**, the process clearly involves more than simply calculated low-density lipoprotein-cholesterol (LDL-C)[6-8]; further elucidation of other causative or involved factors and mechanisms may add to the ability to risk-stratify populations, and it is hoped, individual patients, and improve preventive treatment.

Observations regarding ischemic heart disease began centuries ago; however, modern appreciation of ASCVD's causes and disease risk began with the National Heart Act signed into law in 1948, which established the National Heart Institute and provided a $500,000 grant for a 20-year epidemiologic study of cardiovascular (CV) disease, which became known as the Framingham Heart Study (FHS).[9] The first subject was enrolled 65 years ago when 44% of deaths in the United States were due to ASCVD. The FHS led to the identification of several major ASCVD risk factors, including cigarette smoking, hypertension, and elevated serum cholesterol; family history was added subsequently.

Presented is a brief review of the current state of ASCVD risk assessment and prevention treatment guidelines with attention to limitations that encourage improvement.

ATHEROSCLEROTIC CARDIOVASCULAR DISEASE RISK FACTORS

The major, now termed traditional, risk factors (**Fig. 2**) are the foundation of all ASCVD risk assessment systems or scores and preventive treatment recommendations.[10] Starting with the Framingham Risk Score (FRS), most systems use, almost exclusively, these traditional risk factors. Because decreased high-density lipoprotein-cholesterol (HDL-C) is strongly associated with increased risk of CV events and elevated HDL-C is strongly associated with decreased risk,[11] some scores include it as a positive or negative factor, depending on levels. The INTERHEART Study[12] was a large, international (52 countries), standardized, case-control study evaluating the strength of association between a variety of risk factors and acute MI and whether this association varied by geographic region, ethnic origin, sex, or age. **Box 2** lists 9 risk, or protective factors, which identified almost 90% of those at risk of a first MI, clearly significantly

---

Box 1
Apolipoprotein B particles

Atherogenic (ApoB) lipoproteins
- Very low-density lipoprotein (VLDL)
- Intermediate-density lipoprotein
- LDL
- LDL-P
- Lipoprotein (a)

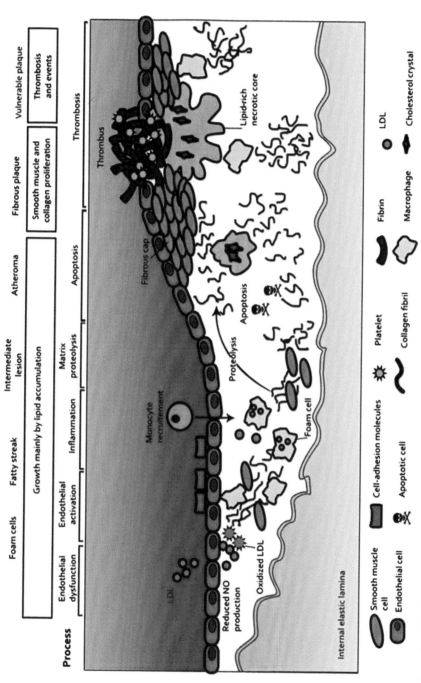

Fig. 1. Genesis and pathophysiology of ASCVD.

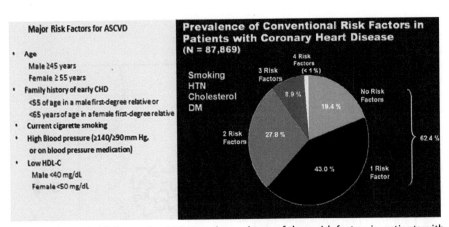

Fig. 2. Traditional risk factors for ASCVD and prevalence of these risk factors in patients with premature CAD; greater than 62% of patient with ASCVD have none or one risk factor. (*Courtesy of* Paul M. Ridker, MD, Boston, MA.)

better than the 50% to 60% most current scoring systems achieve. A variety of nontraditional markers or potential risk factors have been identified; however, evidence of their ability to significantly improve risk prediction, in large groups or populations, remains elusive.[13]

Preventive efforts during the last 30 years have led to significant decreases in ASCVD mortality, nonfatal events, and revascularization.[14] During the same period, the prevalence of risk factors, including hypercholesterolemia, cigarette smoking, and blood pressure (BP), have slightly decreased,[15] with simultaneous increases in the prevalence of obesity, increased body mass index (BMI), increased waist circumference, metabolic syndrome, type II diabetes, and serum triglycerides (TG).[16–18]

Risk factor identification beginning with the FHS may have increased interest in prevention- by the 1970s; however, the statin era clearly has had a dramatic effect, bringing prevention, the ability on a routine basis to decrease CV events, into the modern era and daily clinical practice. Although lifestyle modification has clearly become a linchpin of population prevention, the ability to quickly lower cholesterol, apoB atherogenic lipoproteins, and achieve significant early outcome benefit has helped encourage more

---

Box 2
Risks/protective factors evaluated in the INTERHEART study

- ApoB1/ApoA1 ratio
- Smoking
- Hypertension (self-reported)
- Diabetes
- Abdominal obesity
- Psychosocial factors
- Daily consumption of fruits and vegetables
- Regular alcohol consumption
- Regular physical activity

Collectively, these factors accounted for 90% of the population-attributable risks in men and 94% in women.[12]

aggressive across-the-board prevention efforts. Secondary prevention trials[19] have provided such powerful data that statin treatment is now a universal standard of care. Primary prevention, in patients without known disease but at increased risk, remains somewhat more controversial because of significantly increased number of patients needed to treat to prevent events, potential adverse statin effects and toxicity, and decreased or questionable cost-effectiveness[20] which presents a major question, or perhaps the nexus, of risk versus desirability of treatment. Therefore, there is a significant interest in continuing the search for improved risk factor identification, development of more accurate risk assessment systems, and better preventive treatments.

LIMITATIONS OF CURRENT RISK ASSESSMENT SYSTEMS/SCORES

The acknowledged major risk factors for ASCVD have remained basically unchanged while simultaneously much of CV medicine has not just evolved but been revolutionized. Many do not realize current risk assessment systems and guidelines:

- Identify less than 50% of adults who will develop clinically significant ASCVD,
- Do not identify those in the highest risk group who will have recurrent CV events (residual risk),
- Use 10-year and not lifetime risk (**Fig. 3**)[21] when life expectancy has increased dramatically, therefore discouraging earlier more aggressive prevention efforts,
- Recommend use of ASCVD event cut points to guide treatment; however, no specific cut points for increased risk and events exist,[22]
- Use LDL-C exclusively and do not include a variety of novel non-LDL-C markers because controversy remains regarding whether they improve risk stratification in populations studied.[12,23–25]

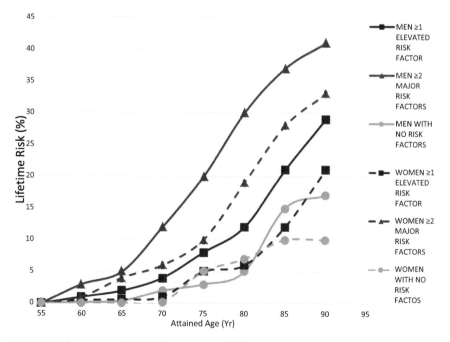

Fig. 3. This figure reveals significant increased lifetime versus 10-year risk of a cardiovascular event in men and women especially with more than 1 traditional risk factor. (*Data from* Berry JD, Dyer A, Cai X, et al. Lifetime risks of cardiovascular disease. N Engl J Med 2012;366:321–9.)

One of the limitations of using only traditional risk factors is a failure to quantify, a basic epidemiologic principle, exposure. For example, exposure to one cigarette a day for a total of a year does not lead to statistically significant increases in the long-term risk of smoking-related illness. However, smoking a pack a day for 20 years would be associated with significantly increased risk. A comprehensive patient history should uncover a more accurate smoking history than the common cursory estimate. Nevertheless, this is not common practice. How can a gross and at times questionably inaccurate estimate of exposure to major risk factors not detrimentally affect individual risk stratification?

A positive family history of ASCVD in first-degree relatives is considered a major risk factor. However, again it is not graded or quantified and not included in the 2013 guideline. Certainly, when confronted with a patient in daily practice, the number of first-degree relatives, their sex and age at disease onset, or particular type of clinical event might influence further patient evaluation and preventive treatment. Increased incidence of ASCVD in a family may have a disproportionate relationship to risk and events, especially in younger individuals.[26,27]

All scores include a history of or treated hypertension as a major factor. However, exposure to systolic hypertension is not quantified via its levels, duration, and adequacy of chronic treatment (**Table 1**). How is the risk of someone with long-term well-controlled BP on one drug versus poorly controlled BP on multiple drugs assessed and compared?

If the role and contribution of each risk factor to events is directly related to exposure, and early and prolonged exposure to atherogenic cholesterol is the proximate or initiating cause of atherosclerosis, why has there not been an attempt to better quantify that relationship?[5,22]

Because the relationship between atherogenic cholesterol and disease is well established, a logical question would be whether LDL-C lowering (apoB, non-HDL-C) earlier in life would delay the development of atherosclerosis and further improve outcomes.[28] Analysis from the 170,000 participants participating in 27 statin trials conducted by the Cholesterol Treatment Trialists Collaboration (CTT)[19] revealed approximately 21% reduction in CVD for every 38.7 mg/dL reduction in LDL-C.[20]

Unfortunately, even with aggressive LDL-C lowering, residual risk for further CV events remains. The mean age at the time of randomization in statin trials evaluated by the CTT group was 63 years. It is not unreasonable to think that LDL-C lowering beginning earlier in life would decrease events and so-called residual risk. Withholding safe treatment of any type until a certain age, reaching a specific absolute risk level (a crude estimate), or until there is evidence of disease seems illogical. In addition, after sustained LDL-C lowering, clinical trial data are consistent with maintained risk reduction for years afterward.[29,30] It would be hard to imagine that better quantification (degree and duration) of a variety of factors, both LDL-C and non-HDL-C, would prove to be a major aid in improving risk stratification.

There are substantial data regarding increased risk in certain ethnic groups. People of south Asian decent especially exhibit increased risk.[31,32] It is accelerated for those who immigrate or are first generation to many industrialized countries.[33] This additional but dramatic effect of ethnicity is rarely considered in risk stratification outside of native countries, even as immigration and worldwide diversity has increased. Is ethnicity worthy of more consideration in the scoring systems?[34]

The basic lipid panel universally used misses as much as 50% of those at risk for ASCVD events. It is now understood that calculated LDL-C is not uncommonly inaccurate in estimating atherogenic cholesterol[35–37] and may occur in a variety of situations, including hypertriglyceridemia, increased waist circumference, metabolic

Table 1
Comparison of variables used in various risk calculation tools

	PROCAM Predicts MI Risk	FRS 2009 CCS Canadian Cholesterol Guidelines	Reynolds Risk Score	Pooled Cohort Equation ACC/ AHA 2013 ASCVD
Age	20–75 y range	Any age in years	Up to age of 80 y	Any age in years
Sex	M/F	M/F	M/F	M/F
Race	Not included	Not included	Not included	• White or other • African American
Smoking[a]	Current nicotine consumption (Y/N)	Smoker or nonsmoker (Y/N)	Smoker or nonsmoker (Y/N)	Smoker or non-smoker (Y/N)
DM[b]	Known DM or FRS ≥120	Diabetic or not (Y/N)	Not included	Diabetic or not (Y/N)
Family history[a]	Positive/negative (1st degree with MI before 60) (Y/N)	Not included	Mother or father have MI before age 60 (Y/N)	Not included
Systolic BP[b]	100–225 mm Hg	Any BP in mm Hg	Any BP in mm Hg	Any BP in mm Hg
Weight	40–120 kg	Not included	Not included	Not included
Height	140–210 cm	Not included	Not included	Not included
Antihypertensive therapy[b]	Receiving therapy or not (Y/N)	Receiving therapy or not (Y/N)	Not included	Receiving therapy or not (Y/N)
Total cholesterol	Not included	Serum levels in mg/dL	Serum levels in mmol or mg/dL	Serum levels in mg/dL
HDL cholesterol	Not included	Serum levels in mg/dL	Serum levels in mmol or mg/dL	Serum levels in mg/dL
hsCRP	Not included	Not included	Serum levels in mg/L	Not included

[a] Not specific to cigarette smoking or amount.
[b] No information on treated/controlled disease versus treated/uncontrolled or duration of controlled/uncontrolled disease.

syndrome, and diabetes (**Table 2**). These situations where LDL-C may not be an accurate reflection of the number of circulating atherogenic particles (apoB, LDL particle number [LDL-P]) can lead to misclassification of risk of patients and therefore failure to appropriately address preventive treatment. Non-HDL-C (total cholesterol [TC] − HDL-C = non-HDL-C) has been recognized as a better risk predictor than LDL-C in a variety of circumstances, especially in women.[4] It correlates better with apoB than LDL-C in many circumstances. Although as noted above, there may have been a modest decrease in overall LDL-C across the population since the FHS began, there has been a significant increase in TG. Even modest elevations in TG can be associated with inaccurate calculation of LDL-C. In the 40 years since the Friedewald Formula (**Box 3**) was developed, adult Americans have steadily increased their weight, waist circumference, BMI, TG, and incidence of cardiometabolic disease. It was anticipated that the new American Heart Association (AHA)/American College of Cardiology (ACC) guideline would recommend non-HDL be used in conjunction with, in addition to, or in

Table 2
Metabolic syndrome*

Measure	Categorical Cut Points
1. Elevated waist circumference	≥40 inches (≥102 cm) in men ≥35 inches (≥88 cm) in women
2. Elevated TG	≥150 mg/dL
3. Reduced HDL-C	<40 mg/dL in men <50 mg/dL women
4. Elevated blood pressure (antihypertensive drug therapy in a patient with a history of hypertension is an alternate indicator)	Systolic ≥130 or diastolic≥85 mm Hg
5. Elevated fasting glucose (drug therapy of elevated glucose is an alternate indicator)	≥100 mg/dL

* The diagnosis of metabolic syndrome requires at least 3 of the above measures.

place of LDL-C in risk assessment and treatment decisions. Some think this failure represents a lost opportunity.

A variety of non-LDL-C lipoprotein, metabolic, and inflammatory markers, although not considered powerful enough to make statistically significant improvements in outcomes in the populations studied, may be useful in a variety of subgroups, including elevated TG, decreased HDL-C, and increased high-sensitivity C-reactive protein (hsCRP). Ridker and colleagues[38] documented significantly increased independent risk of MI and cerebrovascular events or stroke in apparently healthy men secondary to elevated hsCRP (**Fig. 4**), leading to the development of the Reynolds Risk Score.[39]

The prior 2 paragraphs refer to cardiometabolic disease and risk (**Box 4**). The epidemic of insulin resistance, metabolic syndrome, and diabetes is associated with a specific dyslipidemia, including elevated TG, decreased HDL-C, and a proinflammatory/prothrombotic state, increasing the risk of ASCVD events.[17] Sixty-five percent of those with diabetes die from some form of heart disease or stroke. For this reason, National Cholesterol Education (NCEP) Adult Treatment Panel (ATP) III declared diabetes an ASCVD equivalent (**Table 3**).[10]

CLINICAL GUIDELINES

Publication of The Dartmouth Atlas of Cardiovascular Care in 1999,[40] based on a tabulation of where Medicare patients were hospitalized, made clear what many had suspected, that great variations in medical practice, including utilization of CV procedures and interventions, existed around the country. This finding prompted the federal government and third-party payers to begin questioning the indications, justification, and cost for significant amounts of health care delivered. The ACC and AHA working cooperatively were in the vanguard of organizations developing what have become

Box 3
Friedewald formula 1975

LDL-C = TC – HDL-C – TG/5

This assumes a fixed factor of 5 for the ratio of TG to VLDL-C; however, the actual TG:VLDL-C ratio varies significantly across a range of TG and cholesterol levels.

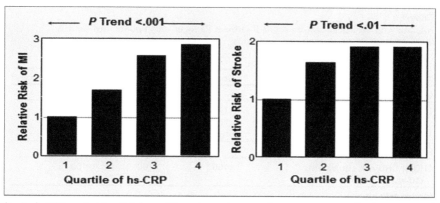

Fig. 4. hsCRP and risk of future MI and cerebrovascular events or stroke in apparently healthy men. (*Data from* Ridker PM, Cushman M, Stampfer MJ, et al. Inflammation, aspirin and the risk of cardiovascular disease in apparently healthy men. N Engl J Med 1997;336:973–9.)

known as practice guidelines or recommendations to assist clinicians in addressing various patient care issues. Treatment guidelines have become increasingly important because the incidence of ASCVD in the population remains high and issues of appropriate and quality care are now paramount. Multiple organizations, especially the National Institutes of Health and the Institute of Medicine, have developed and refined processes to determine what specific guideline efforts are necessary and how to proceed.[41,42] This process includes developing the structure and rules regarding issues such as how to choose professionals knowledgeable and respected enough to lead these efforts and using the best clinical evidence available. Rigorous attention to potential conflicts of interest of all parties involved is now standard procedure.

A host of ways has been developed to collect health care data, study clinical problems, and analyze results. Although during the past 3 decades randomized clinical trials (RCTs) have become the gold standard used in the development of guidelines, this type of robust data is not always available in the quality, quantity, and timeliness needed. Therefore, using a variety of different types/levels of data and analysis as shown in (**Fig. 5**) has been used.

The AHA/ACC clinical guidelines are placed in 3 groups or classifications (**Fig. 6**) but there is a degree of consistency across all guidelines. To help with this process, the levels of evidence used in forming these classifications are also graded. The

---

Box 4
Cardiometabolic risk

- Abdominal obesity
- ↑TG ↓HDL-C
- Insulin resistance
- Metabolic syndrome
- Diabetes
- Proinflammatory
- Prothrombotic

Table 3
National Cholesterol Education Adult Treatment Panel III 2004 update: low-density lipoprotein-cholesterol goals and cut points

Risk Category	LDL-C (mg/dL)		
	Goal	Initiate TLC	Consider Therapy[a]
Very high (NEW)			
CVD + multiple risk factors (especially diabetes), severe/poorly controlled risk factors, metabolic syndrome, or ACS	<100 <70 optional goal	≥100	≥100
High			
CHD or CHD risk equivalents (10-year risk>20%)	<100	≥100	≥100
Moderately high			
2+ risk factors (10-year risk 10%–20%)	<130[b]	≥130	≥130
Moderate			
2+ risk factors (10-year risk <10%)	<130	≥130	≥160
Low			
0–1 risk factor	<160	≥160	≥190

Abbreviations: TLC, therapeutic lifestyle change; ACS, acute coronary syndrome.
 [a] In patients with moderate risk or greater, use therapy to achieve at least a 30%–40% LDL-C reduction.
 [b] Optional goal less than 100 mg/dL.

documents produced undergo multiple levels of careful review and numerous revisions. Although, as expected, these documents sometimes raise questions, concerns, or criticisms, the process is rigorous, depends on extraordinary participation and commitment of all of those involved, and attempts to produce the most comprehensive and appropriate guidelines for the time.

Although clinical guidelines have become a great aid for health care professionals, invariably limitations remain. Evidence-based medicine has become a commonplace mantra in recent years; however, the reality is there are limited amounts of powerful randomized trial data available to support expanding clinical guidelines. Tricoci and

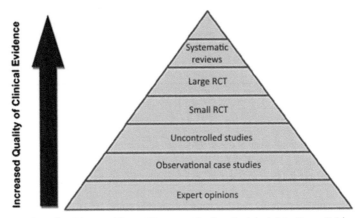

Fig. 5. Hierarchy of evidence. (*From* Therapeutic Goods Administration. Evidence guidelines: guidelines on the evidence required to support indications for listed complementary medicines. Commonwealth of Australia, Department of Health. Version 2.1, July 2014.)

SIZE OF TREATMENT EFFECT

	CLASS I
	Benefit >>> Risk
	Procedure/Treatment
	SHOULD be performed/
	administered
		CLASS IIa
		Benefit >> Risk
		Additional studies with
		focused objectives needed
		IT IS REASONABLE to per-
		form procedure/administer
		treatment
			CLASS IIb
			Benefit ≥ Risk
			Additional studies with broad
			objectives needed; additional
			registry data would be helpful
			Procedure/Treatment
			MAY BE CONSIDERED
				CLASS III *No Benefit*
				or CLASS III *Harm*
				      Procedure/
				      Test Treatment
				COR III: Not No Proven
				No benefit Helpful Benefit
				COR III: Excess Cost Harmful
				Harm w/o Benefit to Patients
				       or Harmful

LEVEL A Multiple populations evaluated* Data derived from multiple randomized clinical trials or meta-analyses	■ Recommendation that procedure or treatment is useful/effective ■ Sufficient evidence from multiple randomized trials or meta-analyses	■ Recommendation in favor of treatment or procedure being useful/effective ■ Some conflicting evidence from multiple randomized trials or meta-analyses	■ Recommendation's usefulness/efficacy less well established ■ Greater conflicting evidence from multiple randomized trials or meta-analyses	■ Recommendation that procedure or treatment is not useful/effective and may be harmful ■ Sufficient evidence from multiple randomized trials or meta-analyses
LEVEL B Limited populations evaluated* Data derived from a single randomized trial or nonrandomized studies	■ Recommendation that procedure or treatment is useful/effective ■ Evidence from single randomized trial or nonrandomized studies	■ Recommendation in favor of treatment or procedure being useful/effective ■ Some conflicting evidence from single randomized trial or nonrandomized studies	■ Recommendation's usefulness/efficacy less well established ■ Greater conflicting evidence from single randomized trial or nonrandomized studies	■ Recommendation that procedure or treatment is not useful/effective and may be harmful ■ Evidence from single randomized trial or nonrandomized studies
LEVEL C Very limited populations evaluated* Only consensus opinion of experts, case studies, or standard of care	■ Recommendation that procedure or treatment is useful/effective ■ Only expert opinion, case studies, or standard of care	■ Recommendation in favor of treatment or procedure being useful/effective ■ Only diverging expert opinion, case studies, or standard of care	■ Recommendation's usefulness/efficacy less well established ■ Only diverging expert opinion, case studies, or standard of care	■ Recommendation that procedure or treatment is not useful/effective and may be harmful ■ Only expert opinion, case studies, or standard of care
Suggested phrases for writing recommendations	should is recommended is indicated is useful/effective/beneficial	is reasonable can be useful/effective/beneficial is probably recommended or indicated	may/might be considered may/might be reasonable usefulness/effectiveness is unknown/unclear/uncertain or not well established	COR III: COR III: No Benefit Harm is not potentially recommended harmful is not indicated causes harm should not be associated with performed/ excess morbid- administered/ ity/mortality other should not be is not useful/ performed/ beneficial/ administered/ effective other
Comparative effectiveness phrases†	treatment/strategy A is recommended/indicated in preference to treatment B treatment A should be chosen over treatment B	treatment/strategy A is probably recommended/indicated in preference to treatment B it is reasonable to choose treatment A over treatment B		

A recommendation with Level of Evidence B or C does not imply that the recommendation is weak. Many important clinical questions addressed in the guidelines do not lend themselves to clinical trials. Even when randomized trials are unavailable, there may be a very clear clinical consensus that a particular test or therapy is useful or effective.

*Data available from clinical trials or registries about the usefulness/efficacy in different subpopulations, such as sex, age, history of diabetes, history of prior myocardial infarction, history of heart failure, and prior aspirin use.

†For comparative-effectiveness recommendations (Class I and IIa; Level of Evidence A and B only), studies that support the use of comparator verbs should involve direct comparisons of the treatments or strategies being evaluated.

Fig. 6. Evaluating and classifying levels of evidence for guideline development. (*From* Goff DC Jr, Lloyd-Jones DM, Bennett G, et al. 2013 ACC/AHA guideline on the assessment of cardiovascular risk: a report of the American College of Cardiology/American Heart Association Task Force on Practice Guidelines. J Am Coll Cardiol 2014;63(25 Pt B):2935–59.)

colleagues[43] published "Scientific Evidence Underlying the ACC/AHA Clinical Practice Guidelines" in February 2009 revealing that most ACC/AHA recommendations are not based on randomized trials (level A) but on lower levels of evidence along with expert opinion and concluded the proportion of recommendations for which there is no conclusive evidence base is actually growing. Neuman and colleagues,[44] in "Durability of Class I American College of Cardiology/American Heart Association Clinical Practice Guideline Recommendations," published earlier last year, note that the approaches previously used by ACC/AHA varied across different guidelines and levels of evidence and have been frequently changed or modified. The 2013 AHA/ACC cholesterol treatment guideline[29] based only on prespecified RCTs and a large meta-analysis may have led to different limitations and concerns. Therefore, when the question arises, sometimes passionately, where is the evidence, one should be prepared for the answer. There may not be adequate powerful data or clear-cut evidence available, and may never be, depending on the situation. This fact only supports how important experience and judgment continue to be in patient care, as recommended in all guidelines produced. An additional factor that appears to produce few comments or suggested future solutions is that a very significant amount of the randomized data used to produce these evidence-based guidelines has come from industry-sponsored trials, with a much smaller contribution from other sources like the National Heart, Lung, and Blood Institute (NHLBI). Whether continued support for these major important efforts is maintained in the current health care environment remains to be seen.

The NCEP ATP III was disseminated in 2002[45] with a brief update in 2004.[42] The medical community was anticipating production of NCEP ATP IV when the NHLBI requested the AHA, ACC, the National Lipid Association (NLA), and other stakeholder organizations to develop a new practice guideline for risk assessment, reduction of CV events, and management of blood cholesterol. This request led to publication of the "2013 AHA/ACC Guideline on the Treatment of Blood Cholesterol to Reduce Atherosclerotic Cardiovascular Risk in Adults."[29] The NLA chose not to participate in this effort. A comprehensive review of the entire process is available in the recent AHA/ACC guideline publication. This process excluded use of a wide variety of information and led to significant modifications in the scope of the guideline compared with the ATP III. This more limited approach and resultant recommendations have met with some discomfort by many health care professionals and stakeholder organizations.

Starting with the FRS (**Fig. 7**), studies have revealed that physicians are poor at estimating absolute individual risk even with easy-to-use formulas that allow rapid calculation based on simple accepted traditional risk factors. The 2013 AHA/ACC Guideline on the Assessment of Cardiovascular Risk panel developed new 10-year risk equations (Pooled Cohort Equations) for a broad US population providing sex- and race-specific estimates for ASCVD events, including coronary heart disease (CHD) and stroke.[29]

There was initial skepticism regarding the predictive accuracy of these new equations but further evaluation seems to justify their use certainly being no less predictive than other systems.[46] They directly address risk for ASCVD in women and African Americans. A downloadable computer and phone application that allows rapid input of information and calculation of 10-year risk is available, thus simplifying the process of obtaining a percentage of absolute risk in individual patients and applying any treatment recommendations.

The new ACC/AHA guideline identifies 4 high-risk groups and recommends high-intensity (group 1) or moderate dose (groups 2–4) statin therapy be initiated (**Table 4**):

1. Secondary prevention in patients with clinical ASCVD,
2. Primary prevention in those with LDL-C of 190 mg/dL or higher,
3. Primary prevention in those with diabetes who are between 40 and 75 years of age with LDL-C 70–189 mg/dL,
4. Primary prevention in patients with an estimated 10-year risk of CV disease of 7.5% or greater who are between 40 and 75 years of age (using the pooled cohort risk assessment equations for calculating 10-year risk).

Guideline development was based on data from specific large RCTs and one meta-analysis. It appears that the panel thought that these data strongly supported the use of statins, that no other drug group or class had unequivocal evidence of outcome benefit and did not support a specific treatment target or goal. Rather, the large amount of data supported treatment in specific conditions and statin doses producing a percentage of LDL-C reduction related to decreased events.[47] Because the treatment goal is statin use (dose) and not a specific level of LDL-C, repeat measurement is recommended only to assess drug adherence once the treatment is initiated. This has received some criticism from various professionals and organizations. The NLA

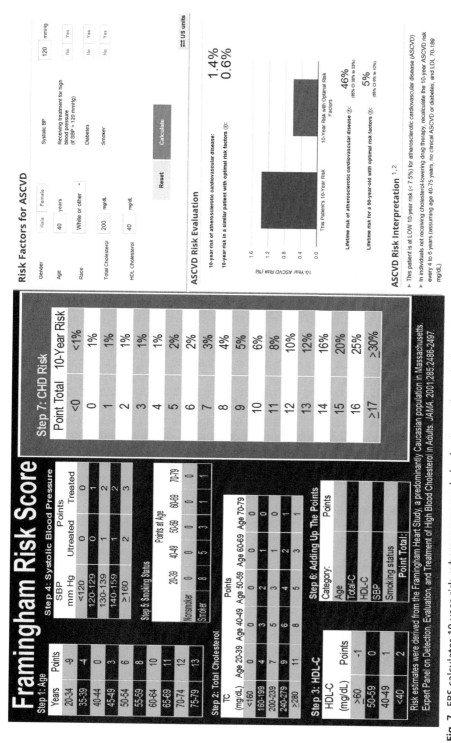

Fig. 7. FRS calculates 10-year risk, whereas new pooled cohort equation calculates 10-year as well as lifetime risk. Note the significant increase in lifetime risk versus 10-year risk (5% vs 46%, respectively) in a patient of 40 years with total cholesterol of 200 mg/dL, HDL 40 mg/dL, nonsmoker, nondiabetic without hypertension. SBP, systolic blood pressure. (Calculator courtesy of ClinCalc.com.)

Table 4
Classification of statins on the bases of their potencies

Statin Therapy		
High-Intensity Daily Dose ↓ LDL-C ≥250%	**Moderate-Intensity Daily Dose** ↓ LDL-C 30 50 <50%	**Low-Intensity Daily Dose** ↓ LDL-C ↓<30%
Atorvastatin 40, 80 mg	Atorvastatin 10, 20 mg	Simvastatin 10 mg
Rosuvastatin 20, 40 mg	Fluvastatin 40 mg bid	Fluvastatin 20–40 mg
	Fluvastatin XL 80 mg	Lovastatin 20 mg
	Lovastation 40 mg	Pitavastatin 1 mg
	Pitavastatin 2–4 mg	Pravastatin 10–20 mg
	Pravastatin 40,80 mg	
	Rosuvastatin 5, 10 mg	
	Simvastatin 20,40 mg	

Individual responses to statin therapy varied in clinical trials should be expected to vary in clinical practice. Values for LDL-C lowering are appropriate averages. Moderate- or high-intensity statin therapy is preferred unless not tolerated.

did not participate in the development of the new AHA/ACC guideline; however, it convened its own Expert Panel and produced "Recommendations for Patient-Centered Management of Dyslipidemia" earlier in 2014 (**Box 5**).[48] As in prior guidelines, this panel used data from randomized trials, meta-analyses as well as epidemiologic, metabolic, genetic data and expert opinion (**Table 5**). Many consider the AHA/ACC effort to be a statin-treatment guideline that fails to address many issues, including the role of family history and other novel non-LDL-C lipids, lipoproteins, and inflammatory factors in risk assessment and treatment. The guideline also does not strongly recommend combination drug treatment for more potent LDL-C lowering and the pivotal importance and role of atherogenic cholesterol (apoB, non-HDL-C) as a treatment target,[49] where the NLA and European Society of Cardiology recommendations do. As such, they are more comprehensive than the critical questions that framed the AHA/ACC effort. Although a variety of trials were unable to reveal outcome benefit with combination lipid-modifying therapy,[50–52] many would argue they did not evaluate the appropriate population (inclusion criteria) necessary.

Many concerns regarding the ACC/AHA guideline have been expressed since publication in November 2013, and some think it may have been a step backward in individualized, patient-centered care. Although extremely safe in all aspects, some think the initial use of moderate- to high-potency statins as an across-the-board approach may expose certain patients to higher risks of side effects and toxicity. The lack of numeric targets, LDL-C, and non-HDL-C and the less than meticulous reassessments recommended may raise a question as to how to insure adequacy and adherence of long-term treatment. Although the intensity of treatment to

Box 5
National Lipid Association 2014 recommendations

Re-screen every 5 years with evaluation of any changes in risk factors, co-morbidities, new secondary causes of dyslipidemia, ASCVD events in first degree relatives, or other changes based on clinical judgment.

—NLA 2014 Recommendations

Table 5
National Lipid Association classifications of cholesterol and triglyceride levels in mg/dL

Non-HDL-C		HDL-C	
<130	Desirable	<40 (men)	Low
<130–159	Above desirable	<50 (women)	Low
160–189	Borderline high		
190–219	High		
≥220	Very high		

LDL-C		TG	
<100	Desirable	<150	Normal
100–129	Above desirable	150–199	Borderline high
130–159	Borderline high	200–499	High
160–189	High	≥500	Very high
≥190	Very high		

Adapted from Jacobson TA, Ito MK, Maki KC, et al. National Lipid Association recommendations for patient-centered management of dyslipidemia: part 1—executive summary. J Clin Lipidol 2014;8(5):473–88.

Box 6
National Lipid Association recommendations

Guiding principles/conclusions

NLA document

1. Elevated level of atherogenic cholesterol, cholesterol carried by apo B-containing lipoprotein particles, is causally related to the development of clinical ASCVD.

2. Reducing elevating levels of apo B will lower ASCVD risk in a direct almost linear fashion.

3. The intensity of risk reduction therapy should be adjusted to the patient's absolute risk for an ASCVD event.

4. For patients in whom lipid drug treatment is indicated, statin treatment is the primary modality for reducing ASCVD risk.

5. Other ASCVD risk factors should be addressed and managed appropriately.

Adapted from Jacobson TA, Ito MK, Maki KC, et al. National Lipid Association recommendations for patient-centered management of dyslipidemia: part 1—executive summary. J Clin Lipidol 2014;8(5):473–88.

Box 7
National Lipid Association cholesterol (lipid panel) screening and surveillance of ASCVD risk

- Children (<13 years old) of parents with premature ASCVD or familial hypercholesterolemia

- Postpubescent (>13 years old) obtain routinely

- Adults greater than 20 years old and every 5 years after in those without multiple ASCVD risk factors and LDL-C less than 130 mg/dL, NLA 2014 less than 190 mg/dL, ACC/AHA 2013 (should include appropriate overall health assessment and ASCVD risk stratification)

Table 6
Comparison between various cholesterol treatment guidelines

	EAS/ESC	AHA/ACC	Canadian Society
Secondary prevention	Treat with a target LDL-C <70 mg/dL (<1.8 mmol/L), or at least 50% reduction	Treat with no particular target. High-intensity statin to reduce LDL-C by 50%	Treat with statins with target goals of ≥50% reduction in LDL-C or to ≤2 mmol/L, OR alternate goals of ApoB ≤0.8 mmol/L or non-HDL ≤2.6 mmol/L
Statin intolerance in secondary prevention	Reduce statin dose, consider combination therapy	Moderate or low-dose statin, consider combination therapy	Reinitiation trial, reduce dose; consider combination therapy
Primary prevention LDL >190 mg/dL (>4.9 mmol/L)	Target LDL-C <100 mg/dL (<2.5 mmol/L). If target cannot be reached, maximal reduction of LDL-C using appropriate drug combinations in tolerated doses	High-intensity statin therapy, aimed at achieving at least 50% reduction of LDL-C. If 50% reduction cannot be achieved, consider additional therapy	Low risk <10% FRS: treat if LDL-C ≥193 mg/d (>5 mmol/L) with reduction of >50% Intermediate risk >10 to <20% FRS: treat if LDL-C ≥135 mg/d (>3.5 mmol/L), OR if LDL-C is <135 mg/dL but has ApoB ≥46 mg/dL (1.2 mmol/L) or non-HDL-C is ≥166 mg/dL (4.6 mmol/L) with goal of ≥50% reduction in LDL-C or to <2 mmol/L or ApoB ≤0.8 mmol/L or non-HDL ≤2.6 mmol/L
Primary prevention in diabetes	Diabetes with other risk factors or organ damage: target LDL-C = 70 mg/dL (1.8 mmol/L), or at least 50% reduction. Uncomplicated diabetes: target LDL-C 100 mg/dL (<2.5 mmol/L)	Diabetes with high risk: high-intensity statin therapy. Diabetes with low risk: moderate-intensity statin therapy	Diabetes of >15 y and age >30 y OR any age above 40 y with the same goals as in secondary prevention

	SCORE = 5% risk of fatal CVD: target 100 mg/dL (<2.5 mmol/L)	Total risk for CVD event >7.5%: Moderate- to high-intensity statin therapy. Risk 5%–7.5% risk of CVD event: moderate-intensity statin therapy	FRS ≥20% for fatal CVD: Target goal of ≥50% reduction in LDL-C or to ≤2 mmol/L, OR alternate goals of ApoB ≤0.8 mmol/L or non-HDL-C ≤2.6 mmol/L
Primary prevention high risk			
Risk calculators	SCORE (Systemic Coronary Risk Estimation)	Pooled cohort risk calculator	Framingham risk calculator
Monitoring	LFTs: before initiation, 8 wk after or after any increase in dose, annually thereafter if LFTs <3× ULN CK: Baseline, no need afterward unless symptomatic Lipid profile: before initiation of therapy, at least 2 measurements with an interval of 1–12 wk, then 8 (±4) wk after start of drug or after the adjustment in dose of drug until within target range, and then annually afterward	LFTs: before initiation, then only of clinically warranted CK: No baseline levels, afterward only if clinically warranted Lipid profile: before initiation of therapy, after 6–12 wk only to assess the compliance	LFTs: before initiation, then only if clinically warranted CK: before initiation, afterward only if clinically warranted Lipid profile: before initiation of therapy
Nonstatin drugs	If target cannot be reached with statin, drug combination may be considered	If 50% reduction is not reached, drug combination may be considered	If target cannot be reached with statin, drug combination may be considered

Abbreviations: CK, creatine kinase; LFT, liver function studies; ULN, upper limit of normal.

reduce ASCVD events should be tailored to a patient's absolute risk, the 10-year risk has continued to be used as an arbitrary cut point for treatment. However, the process and manifestations of ASCVD have no cut points. It is a progressive process with risk increasing, as more risk factors are identified, time and age. Ten-year risk remains an arbitrary determination and allows criticism of the guideline as not being individual but population based. In fact, the document notes "moderate evidence supports the use of statins for primary prevention in individuals with 5%–7.5% 10-year ASCVD risk with LDL-C 70–189 mg/dL." This half-hearted statement does not encourage treatment of many patients who will develop ASCVD during their lives. The authors think it is time to consider the much greater lifetime risk in both men and women as a more appropriate patient-centered approach, although many patients will again be missed before their development of clinically significant disease.

The recent NLA recommendation for the treatment of dyslipidemia[49] proposed several guiding principles (**Boxes 6** and **7**) that may not be greatly different than the ACC/AHA guideline; however, they make a strong statement regarding the role of atherogenic apoB lipoproteins and its measurement and utilization rather than the exclusive use of LDL-C with its limitations in today's population and changing risk spectrum. **Table 6** compares 3 different risk scores most noted for similarities, limited risk stratification strategies and treatment recommendations, than any significant differences.

The new NLA recommendations[48] do address the issues of when to consider using other non-LDL-C risk factors or markers (**Box 8**).

Many health care professionals seem to think ASCVD risk assessment/stratification and treatment recommendations are a settled issue. However, careful evaluation reveals the following: current systems are outdated; a population is not patient centric; and the current systems fail to identify a large percentage of those at risk of ASCVD and events and appear to discourage aggressive prevention treatment strategies. The authors would recommend the following:

- Embracing a more individual or patient-centered approach to risk assessment with more comprehensive and accurate risk factor evaluation,
- Utilizing non-LDL-C markers based on individual risk assessment when appropriate,

---

Box 8
National Lipid Association recommendations on non-LDL-C risk factors or markers

Advanced lipoprotein/biomarker analysis: when to consider

- >5% 10-year ASCVD risk (previously known as intermediate risk)
- ASCVD without significantly elevated LDL-C
- Low HDL-C
- Elevated inflammatory factor
- Metabolic syndrome MS/diabetes mellitus (DM)
- Very strong family history in first-degree relatives
- Active cigarette smoker
- Discordance between presence of ASCVD, age, and lack of multiple risk factors (when something does not make sense)

Adapted from Jacobson TA, Ito MK, Maki KC, et al. National Lipid Association recommendations for patient-centered management of dyslipidemia: part 1—executive summary. J Clin Lipidol 2014;8(5):473–88.

- Using preventive treatment strategies, including pharmacologic intervention, when lifetime and 10-year risk appear discordant,
- Employing a broader use of apoB and non-HDL-C, the total atherogenic burden, versus LDL-C in determining treatment,
- Consider continuing to use treatment targets and more attentive follow-up in specific patients with known disease who you may consider to be at greater risk of recurrent or residual CV events, rather than a fixed-dose strategy with follow-up to determine adherence only.

REFERENCES

1. Lloyd-Jones D, Adams R, Carnethon M, et al. Heart disease and stroke statistics—2009 update: a report from the American Heart Association Statistics Committee and Stroke Statistics Subcommittee. Circulation 2009;119(3):480–6.
2. Enos WF, Holmes RH, Beyer J. Coronary disease among United States soldiers killed in action in Korea: preliminary report. JAMA 1953;552:1090–3.
3. Berenson GS, Srinivasan SR, Bao W, et al. Association between multiple cardiovascular risk factors and atherosclerosis in children and young adults. N Engl J Med 1998;338(23):1650–6. Available at: www.nejm.org. Accessed July 21, 2014.
4. Smith SC, Allen J, Blair SN, et al. AHA/ACC guidelines for secondary prevention for patients with coronary and other atherosclerotic vascular disease: 2006 update: endorsed by the National Heart and Lung and Blood Institute. Circulation 2006;113:2363–72.
5. Tabas I, William KJ, Koren J. Subendothelial lipoprotein retention as the initiating process in atherosclerosis: update and therapeutic implications. Circulation 2007;116:1832–44.
6. Libby P, Ridker PM. Inflammation and atherothrombosis: from population biology and bench research to clinical practice. J Am Coll Cardiol 2006;48:A33–46.
7. Libby P. Inflammation in atherosclerosis. Nature 2002;420:868–74.
8. Libby P, Aikawa M. Stabilization of atherosclerotic plaques: new mechanisms and clinical targets. Nat Med 2002;8:1257–62.
9. Dawber TR, Meadors GF, Moore FE Jr. Epidemiological approaches to heart disease: the Framingham Study. Am J Public Health 1951;41:279–86.
10. Wilson PW, D'Agostino RB, Levy D, et al. Prediction of coronary heart disease using risk factor categories. Circulation 1998;97:1837–47.
11. Kannel W. High-density lipoproteins: epidemiologic profile and risks of coronary artery disease. Am J Cardiol 1983;52:9B–12B.
12. Yusuf S, Hawken S, Ounpuu S, et al. Effect of potentially modifiable risk factors associated with myocardial infarction in 52 countries (the INTERHEART study): case-control study. Lancet 2004;364(9438):937–52.
13. Melander O, Newton-Cheh C, Almgren P, et al. Novel and conventional biomarkers for prediction of incident cardiovascular events in the community. JAMA 2009;302:49–57.
14. American Heart Association. Heart disease & stroke statistics—2010 update. A report from the American Heart Association. Dallas (TX): American Heart Association; 2010.
15. Evans A, Tolonen H, Hense HW, et al, WHO MONICA Project. Trends in coronary risk factors in the WHO MONICA project. Int J Epidemiol 2001;30:S35–40.
16. The SEARCH for Diabetes in Youth Study Group. Incidence of diabetes in youth in the United States. JAMA 2007;297:2716–24.

17. Mokdad AH, Ford ES, Bowman BA, et al. Prevalence of obesity, diabetes, and obesity-related health risk factors, 2001. JAMA 2003;289:76–9.
18. Adult Treatment Panel III. Executive summary of the third report of the National Cholesterol Education Program (NCEP) Expert Panel on detection, evaluation, and treatment of high blood cholesterol in adults. JAMA 2001;285:2486–97.
19. Cholesterol Treatment Trialists Collaboration. Efficacy of cholesterol-lowering treatment: prospective meta-analysis of data from 90,056 patients in 14 randomized trials and statins. Lancet 2005;366:1267–78.
20. Mills EJ, Rachlis B, WU P, et al. Primary prevention of cardiovascular mortality and events with statin treatments: a network meta-analysis involving more than 65,000 patients. J Am Coll Cardiol 2008;52:1769–81.
21. Berry JD, Dyer A, Cai X, et al. Lifetime risks of cardiovascular disease. N Engl J Med 2012;366:321–9.
22. Sachdeva A, Cannon CP, Deedwania PC, et al. Lipid levels in patients hospitalized with coronary artery disease: an analysis of 136,905 hospitalizations in Get With The Guidelines. Am Heart J 2009;157(1):111–7.
23. Parish S, Peto R, Palmer A, et al. The joint effects of apolipoprotein B, apolipoprotein A$_1$, LDL cholesterol, and HDL cholesterol on risk: 3510 cases of acute myocardial infarction and 9805 controls. Eur Heart J 2009;30:2137–46.
24. Willeit P, Kiechl S, Kronenberg F, et al. Discrimination and net reclassification of cardiovascular risk with lipoprotein(a): prospective 15-year outcomes in the Bruneck Study. J Am Coll Cardiol 2014;64:851–60.
25. Morris PB, Wright RF. Transitioning from population to individualized preventative cardiology. Res Rep Clin Cardiol 2013;4:55–9.
26. Berenson GS, Srinivasan SR, Bao W, et al. Association between multiple cardiovascular risk factors and atherosclerosis in children and young adults. N Engl J Med: Available at: www.njem.org. Accessed July 21, 2014.
27. Wilson PW, Garrison RJ, Castelli WP, et al. Prevalence of coronary heart disease in Framingham offspring study: role of lipoprotein cholesterols. J Am Coll Cardiol Available at: http://www.ncbi.nlm.nih.gov/pubmed/7416024. Accessed August 18, 2014.
28. Ference BA, Jahajan N. The role of early LDL lowering to prevent the onset of atherosclerotic disease. Curr Atheroscler Rep 2013;15:312.
29. Stone NJ, Robinson J, Lichtenstein AH, et al. 2013 ACC/AHA guideline on the treatment of blood cholesterol to reduce atherosclerotic cardiovascular risk in adults: a report of the American College of Cardiology/American Heart Association Task Force on Practice Guidelines. J Am Coll Cardiol 2013;63:2889–934.
30. Martin SS, Blumenthal RS, Miller M. LDL cholesterol: the lower the better. Med Clin North Am 2012;96:13–26.
31. Enas EA, Yusuf S, Mehta JL. Prevalence of coronary artery disease in Asian Indians. Am J Cardiol 1992;70(9):945–9.
32. Tillin T, Hughes A, Mayet J. The relationship between metabolic risk factors and incident cardiovascular disease in Europeans, South Asians and African Carribeans: SABRE (Southall and Brent Revisited)—a prospective population-based study. J Am Coll Cardiol 2013;61(17):1778–86.
33. Enas EA, Garg A, Davidson MA. Coronary heart disease and its risk factors in first-generation immigrant Asian Indians to the United States of America. Indian Heart J 1996;48(4):343–53.
34. Gupta M, Singh N, Verma S. South Asians and cardiovascular risk: what clinicians should know. Circulation Available at: http://circ.ahajournals.org/content/113/25/e924. Accessed June 12, 2014.

35. Martin SS, Blaha MJ, Elshazly BE, et al. Friedewald-estimated versus directly measured low-density lipoprotein cholesterol and treatment implications. J Am Coll Cardiol 2013;62(8):732-9.
36. Kilgore M, Muntner P, Woolley JM, et al. Discordance between high non-HDL cholesterol and high LDL-cholesterol among US adults. J Clin Lipidol 2014;8:86-93.
37. Martin SS, Blaha MJ, Elshazly MD, et al. Comparison of a novel method vs the Friedewald equation for estimating low-density lipoprotein cholesterol levels from the standard lipid profile. JAMA 2013;310(19):2061-8.
38. Ridker PM, Cushman M, Stampfer MJ, et al. Inflammation, aspirin and the risk of cardiovascular disease in apparently healthy men. N Engl J Med 1997;336: 973-9.
39. Ridker PM, Buring JE, Rifai N, et al. Development and validation of improved algorithms for assessment of global cardiovascular risk in women: the Reynolds Risk Score. JAMA 2007;297:611-9.
40. Wennberg DE, Birkmeyer JD, Birkmeyer NJ, et al. The Dartmouth atlas of cardiovascular health care. Chicago: AHA Press; 1999.
41. Graham R, Mancher M, Wolman DM, et al, Institute of Medicine. Clinical practice guidelines we can trust. Washington, DC: National Academies Press; 2011.
42. Gibbons GH, Shurin SB, Mensha GA, et al. Refocusing the agenda on cardiovascular guidelines: an appropriate announcement from the National Heart, Lung, and Blood Institute. Circulation 2013;128:1713-5.
43. Tricoci P, Allen JM, Kramer JM, et al. Scientific evidence underlying the ACC/AHA clinical practice guidelines. JAMA 2009;301:831.
44. Neuman MD, Goldstein JN, Cirullo MA, et al. Durability of Class I American College of Cardiology/American Heart Association clinical practice guideline recommendations. JAMA 2014;311(20):2092-100.
45. National Cholesterol Education Program, National Heart, Lung, and Blood Institute, National Institutes of Health. Detection, evaluation, and treatment of high blood cholesterol in adults (Adult treatment panel III) Final report. NIH Publication No. 2-5215. Bethesda (MD): National Cholesterol Education Program, National Heart, Lung, and Blood Institute, National Institutes of Health; 2002.
46. Karmann KN, Goff DC, Ning H, et al. A systematic examination of the 2013 ACC/AHA pooled cohort risk assessment tool for atherosclerotic cardiovascular disease. J Am Coll Cardiol 2014;64(10):959-68.
47. Smith SS, Grundy MS. 2013 ACC/AHA guideline recommends fixed-dose strategies instead of targeted goals to lower cholesterol. J Am Coll Cardiol 2014;64(6): 601-12.
48. Jacobson TA, Ito MK, Maki KC, et al. National Lipid Association recommendations for patient-centered management of dyslipidemia: part 1—executive summary. J Clin Lipidol 2014;8(5):473-88.
49. Boekholdt S, Hovingh GK, Mora S, et al. Very low levels of atherogenic lipoproteins and the risk for cardiovascular events. J Am Coll Cardiol 2014;64(5):485-94.
50. The ACCORD Study Group. Effects of combination lipid therapy in type 2 diabetes mellitus. N Engl J Med 2010;362:1563-74.
51. The AIM-HIGH Investigators. Niacin in patients with low HDL cholesterol levels receiving intensive statin therapy. N Engl J Med 2011;365:2255-67.
52. The HPS2-THRIVE Collaborative Group. Effects of extended-release niacin with laropiprant in high-risk patients. N Engl J Med 2014;371:203-12.

2014 Guideline for the Management of High Blood Pressure (Eighth Joint National Committee): Take-Home Messages

Umar Farooq, MD, MS*, Sunita G. Ray, MD

KEYWORDS

- JNC8 • High blood pressure • Blood pressure goals • Blood pressure treatment

KEY POINTS

- For patients younger than 60 years, the goal blood pressure (BP) is less than 140/90 mm Hg; for patients older than 60 years, the goal BP is less than 150/90 mm Hg.
- For patients with diabetes mellitus and patients with chronic kidney disease (CKD), the goal BP is less than 140/90 mm Hg.
- In nonblack patients with or without diabetes, initial drug-class should include a thiazide-type diuretic, calcium channel blocker (CCB), angiotensin-converting enzyme (ACE) inhibitor, or angiotensin receptor blocker (ARB).
- In black patients with or without diabetes, initial drug-class should include a thiazide-type diuretic or CCB.
- All patients with CKD should receive an ACE inhibitor or ARB as starting or add-on therapy to improve renal outcomes.

High blood pressure (BP) is one of the most common conditions treated in primary care settings worldwide. It is an important preventable condition that leads to morbidity and mortality if not diagnosed timely and/or treated appropriately.[1–3]

The Eighth Joint National Committee (JNC 8) used rigorous evidence-based systematic review of the literature using only randomized control trials (RCTs) to develop evidence statements and recommendations for BP treatment.[4] This report summarizes the key recommendation made by JNC 8 for hypertension management and also highlights important differences from the previous recommendations.

Division of Nephrology, Penn State College of Medicine, Hershey Medical Center, 500 University Drive, Hershey, PA 17033, USA
* Corresponding author. Division of Nephrology, Penn State College of Medicine, Hershey Medical Center, 500 University Drive, Mail Code H040, Hershey, PA 17033.
E-mail address: ufarooq@hmc.psu.edu

Med Clin N Am 99 (2015) 733–738
http://dx.doi.org/10.1016/j.mcna.2015.02.004
0025-7125/15/$ – see front matter © 2015 Elsevier Inc. All rights reserved.

In contrast to JNC 7 guidelines,[5] the 2014 Hypertension Guidelines focus on 3 highest-ranked clinical questions related to hypertension management:

a. BP threshold at which pharmacologic therapy should be initiated
b. Specific BP goal to improve outcomes
c. Comparative benefit and harms on health outcomes using various antihypertensive drug classes

Based on patient age, ethnicity, and comorbid conditions, the following are the summarized recommendations from the JNC 8 for hypertension management.[4]

TREATMENT INITIALIZATION AND GOALS
General Population: Age 60 Years or Older

For the general population aged 60 years or older, it was recommended to start pharmacologic treatment to lower systolic BP (SBP) less than 150 mm Hg and diastolic BP (DBP) less than 90 mm Hg. Additionally, there was no need to adjust treatment if it achieves lower than target SBP levels without being associated with any adverse effects or the quality of life.

General Population: Age Younger Than 60 Years

In this patient age group, pharmacologic treatment is recommended to lower DBP to a goal of less than 90 mm Hg and SBP to a goal of less than 140 mm Hg. In age groups of 30 to 59 years, it is even more important to control DBP to lower than 90 mm Hg.

General Population: Age 18 Years or Older with Diabetes or Chronic Kidney Disease

In this patient population, pharmacologic treatment is also recommended to lower SBP to a goal of less than 140 mm Hg and DBP to a goal of less than 90 mm Hg.

TREATMENT DRUGS OF CHOICE
General Nonblack Population

For the general nonblack population with or without diabetes, recommended initial drugs are the following: thiazide-type diuretic, calcium channel blocker (CCB), angiotensin-converting enzyme inhibitor (ACEI), or angiotensin receptor blocker (ARB).

General Black Population

For the general black population with or without diabetes, initial antihypertensive treatment should include a thiazide-type diuretic or CCB.

General Population: Age 18 Years or Older with Chronic Kidney Disease

Regardless of race or diabetes status, patients with chronic kidney disease (CKD) and hypertension should have ACEI or ARB as initial or add-on treatment to improve kidney functions.

As compared with JNC 7, the current guidelines suggest relaxation of aggressive target BP thresholds in older patients and in patients younger than 60 with diabetes and CKD. Another important consideration is that JNC 7 guidelines mainly defined hypertension and prehypertension, whereas current guidelines focus more on thresholds for pharmacologic treatment.

The JNC 8 panel does not recommend thiazide-type diuretics as initial drug of choice in most patients. In the general nonblack population, it recommends selection among 4 specific classes of medication as initial drug of choice: ACEI, ARB, CCB, or thiazide-type diuretic. For the black population, it recommends 2 medication classes as initial drug of choice: thiazides or CCB.

The JNC 8 also recommends dosing of various antihypertensive medications used in outcome trials and noted that the doses should be adequate to achieve results similar to those seen in RCTs. **Table 1** summarizes the recommended doses.

It is important to note that β-blockers are no longer recommended for initial therapy because they may offer less protection against stroke in one study[6] and other studies showed similar efficacy of a β-blocker compared with the other 4 recommended classes of drugs. Caution should be used when applying recommendations to nonhypertensive patient populations with heart failure and coronary artery disease, as the RCTs limited to this particular subpopulation were not reviewed in JNC 8.

The investigators of JNC 8 noted paucity of good-quality or fair-quality RCT data comparing the 4 recommended classes of drugs with other commonly used antihypertensives. The JCN 8 panel does not recommend use of the following drug classes as

Table 1
Evidence-based dosing of medications

Antihypertensive Medication	Initial Dose	Target Dose in Randomized Controlled Trials and Number of Doses per day
Angiotensin-converting enzyme inhibitors		
Captopril	50 mg	150–200 mg twice a day
Enalapril	5 mg	20 mg in 1-2 doses per day
Lisinopril	10 mg	40 mg daily
Angiotensin receptor blockers		
Eprosartan	400 mg	600–800 mg in 1-2 doses per day
Candesartan	4 mg	12–32 mg daily
Losartan	50 mg	100 mg in 1-2 doses per day
Valsartan	40–80 mg	160–320 mg daily
Irbesartan	75 mg	300 mg daily
Beta-blockers		
Atenolol	25–50 mg	100 mg daily
Metoprolol	50 mg	100–200 mg in 1-2 doses per day
Calcium channel blockers		
Amlodipine	2.5 mg	10 mg daily
Diltiazem extended release	120–180 mg	360 mg daily
Nitrendipine	10 mg	20 mg in 1-2 doses per day
Thiazide-type diuretics		
Bendroflumethiazide	5 mg	10 mg daily
Chlorthalidone	12.5 mg	12.5–25 mg daily
Hydrochlorothiazide	12.5–25 mg	25–100 mg in 1-2 doses per day
Indapamide	1.25 mg	1.25–2.5 mg daily

Table 2
Three suggested strategies to dose the blood pressure (BP) medications
Strategy A	Maximize first medication before adding second and third from the list (thiazide, calcium channel blocker [CCB], angiotensin-converting enzyme inhibitor [ACEI], or angiotensin receptor blocker [ARB]). Avoid both ACEI and ARB together. Titrate each drug to maximum recommended dose to achieve goal BP before adding another medication.
Strategy B	Add second medication before reaching maximum dose of first medication. Titrate both drugs up to the maximum recommended doses to achieve goal BP. If goal BP is not achieved with 2 drugs, select a third drug from the list (thiazide, CCB, ACEI, or ARB). Titrate the third drug up to the maximum recommended dose to achieve goal BP.
Strategy C	Start with 2 medication classes separately or as fixed-dose combinations. Some committee members recommend starting with ≥2 drugs when systolic BP (SBP) is >160 mm Hg and/or diastolic BP (DBP) is >100 mm Hg, or if SBP is >20 mm Hg above goal and/or DBP is >10 mm Hg above goal. If goal BP is not achieved with 2 drugs, select a third drug from the list (thiazide, CCB, ACEI, or ARB). Titrate the third drug up to the maximum recommended dose to achieve goal BP.

first-line therapy: dual α1-blocking + β-blocking agents (eg, carvedilol), direct vasodilators (eg, hydralazine), central α2-adrenergic agonists (eg, clonidine), aldosterone receptor antagonists (eg, spironolactone), adrenergic neuronal depleting agents (reserpine), and loop diuretics (eg, furosemide).

Additionally, the JNC 8 panel also recommended 3 strategies to uptitrate the dose of medications to achieve the sustained control of BP (**Tables 2** and **3**). This includes

Table 3		
Strategies to dose and titrate antihypertensive drugs		
A	B	C
Maximize first medication before adding second.	Add second medication before reaching maximum dose of first medication.	Start with 2 medication classes separately or as fixed-dose combinations.
If goal BP not achieved		
• Reinforce compliance with medication and lifestyle. • For strategies A and B, add and titrate thiazide-type diuretic or angiotensin-converting enzyme inhibitor (ACEI) or angiotensin receptor blocker (ARB) or calcium channel blocker (CCB) (use medication class not previously selected and avoid combined use of ACEI and ARB). • For strategy C, titrate doses of initial medications to maximum.		
If goal BP not achieved		
• Reinforce compliance with medication and lifestyle. • Add and titrate thiazide-type diuretic or ACEI or ARB or CCB (use medication class not previously selected and avoid combined use of ACEI and ARB).		
If goal BP not achieved		
• Reinforce compliance with medication and lifestyle. • Add additional medication class (eg, β-blocker, aldosterone antagonist, or others) and/or refer to physician with expertise in hypertension management.		

Table 4
Summary recommendations from JNC 8

Patient Subgroup	Target SBP (mm Hg)	Target DBP (mm Hg)
Age ≥60 y	<150	<90
Age <60 y	<140	<90
Age >18 y with CKD	<140	<90
Age >18 y with diabetes	<140	<90

General population (nonblack)
• Thiazides, CCB, ACEI, or ARB initially
General population (black)
• Thiazides or CCB initially
Chronic kidney disease
• Treatment should include ACEI or ARB
Adjust therapy after 1 month if BP goal not achieved.
Do not use ACEI or ARB together.
If patients need >3 drugs, refer to hypertension specialist.

Abbreviations: ACEI, angiotensin-converting enzyme inhibitor; ARB, angiotensin receptor blocker; CCB, calcium channel blocker; CKD, chronic kidney disease; DBP, diastolic blood pressure; JNC 8, Eighth Joint National Committee; SBP, systolic blood pressure.

either maximizing doses of individual drugs sequentially or combining several drug classes at lower doses.

SUMMARY

The JNC 8 guidelines focus on the 3 highest-ranked clinical questions that include BP thresholds for starting therapy, specific BP goals, and risks and benefits of specific antihypertensive drugs (**Table 4**). Only RCT data were used and the JNC 8 panel did not include observational studies, systematic reviews, or meta-analyses. The investigators also suggested that benefit of lowering BP to less than 140/90 is not clear. Lifestyle modifications, such as healthy diet, regular exercise, and weight control, were considered very important for all patients with hypertension. These recommendations are not alternatives for clinical judgment, and decisions about medical care must be individualized to each patient.

REFERENCES

1. Ong KL, Cheung BM, Man YB, et al. Prevalence, awareness, treatment, and control of hypertension among United States adults 1999–2004. Hypertension 2007; 49(1):69–75.
2. Go AS, Mozaffarian D, Roger VL, et al. Heart disease and stroke statistics—2014 update: a report from the American Heart Association. Circulation 2014;129: e28–292.
3. Beckett NS, Peters R, Fletcher AE, et al. Treatment of hypertension in patients 80 years of age or older. N Engl J Med 2008;358(18):1887–98.
4. James PA, Oparil S, Carter BL, et al. 2014 evidence-based guideline for the management of high blood pressure in adults: report from the panel members appointed to the Eighth Joint National Committee (JNC 8). JAMA 2014;311(5): 507–20.

5. Chobanian AV, Bakris GL, Black HR, et al. The seventh report of the joint national committee on prevention, detection, evaluation, and treatment of high blood pressure: the JNC 7 report. JAMA 2003;289(19):2560–72.

6. Dahlof B, Devereux RB, Kjeldsen SE, et al. Cardiovascular morbidity and mortality in the Losartan Intervention For Endpoint reduction in hypertension study (LIFE): a randomised trial against atenolol. Lancet 2002;359(9311): 995–1003.

How to Follow Patients with Mitral and Aortic Valve Disease

 CrossMark

Blase Carabello, MD

KEYWORDS

- Mitral valve • Aortic valve • Valvular heart disease • Myocardium

KEY POINTS

- The onset of symptoms for any valvular heart disease is ominous.
- Echocardiography is the mainstay of diagnosis.
- Surgery to correct valve disease must occur before irreversible left ventricular damage has occurred and the indicators for such damage must be recognized.

GENERAL PRINCIPLES

All valvular heart diseases (VHDs) place a hemodynamic load on the left ventricle (LV) and/or right ventricle (RV) that, if severe, prolonged, and untreated, damages the myocardium, leading to heart failure and death. Because all VHDs are mechanical problems, definitive therapy almost always (except for secondary mitral regurgitation [MR]) requires a mechanical solution in the form of valve repair or replacement. As with other realms of medicine, these beneficial therapies have inherent risks, including the risk of surgical or percutaneous valve replacement and the risks of valve prostheses, which include structural failure, thromboembolism, and infection. The goals of following patients with VHDs are to assess disease severity and to time mechanical intervention to optimize this risk/benefit ratio. In order to do this, mechanical therapy must occur early enough in the course of disease to avoid hemodynamically mediated myocardial damage and/or sudden death but late enough to avoid unnecessary procedures and unneeded exposure to the risks of prosthetic heart valves. Although it is not perfect, clinical science has evolved so that careful patient surveillance can fairly accurately time this optimum moment for intervention, which is the topic of this article.

AORTIC STENOSIS

Relationship of Pathophysiology to Symptoms

Although rheumatic heart disease is a common cause of aortic stenosis (AS) in developing countries, in developed countries leaflet calcification resulting from an active

Department of Cardiology, Beth Israel Medical Center, 350 East 17th Street, 5th Floor, Baird Hall, New York, NY 10003, USA
E-mail address: bcarabello@chpnet.org

Med Clin N Am 99 (2015) 739–757
http://dx.doi.org/10.1016/j.mcna.2015.02.005
0025-7125/15/$ – see front matter © 2015 Elsevier Inc. All rights reserved.

medical.theclinics.com

inflammatory process akin to atherosclerosis is the usual cause of AS.[1] Calcified nodules accrue on the aortic side of the valve causing it to stiffen, reducing its orifice area (**Fig. 1**).[2] Little hemodynamic consequence occurs as valve area decreases from its normal 3.0 cm² to one-half that area. However, as orifice area decreases further, left ventricular pressure must increase to drive output past the narrowed valve. At an orifice area of 1.0 cm², a mean pressure gradient of 25 mm Hg typically exists between the LV and the aorta. At a valve area of 0.7 cm², the gradient increases to 50 mm Hg and at a valve area of 0.5 cm² the typical pressure gradient is 100 mm Hg. This pressure overload in turn causes the LV to develop concentric LV hypertrophy (LVH), which is usually viewed initially as a compensatory mechanism.[3] Left ventricular afterload is often described as wall stress (σ), according to the Laplace law, which states that $\sigma = P \times r/2h$, where P is LV pressure, r is LV radius, and h is LV thickness. As the pressure term increases in the Laplace numerator it can be offset by increased thickness in the denominator, maintaining normal afterload and thus normal ejection fraction (EF). However, LVH also results in pathologic consequences and symptoms. The classic symptoms of AS are angina, syncope, and dyspnea. As shown in **Fig. 2**, symptom onset dramatically changes the untreated natural history from a risk of death of less than 1.0% per year in the absence of symptoms to about 25% per year after symptom onset. In turn, symptom onset is linked to hypertrophy.[3,4] Wall thickening may outpace capillary growth, resulting in reduced coronary blood flow reserve potentiating the onset of the symptom of angina.[5,6] Because it takes greater distending pressure to fill a thicker chamber, concentric LVH inherently causes diastolic dysfunction, further exacerbated when collagen content increases as the disease process progresses.[7,8] Systolic function is also compromised in advanced AS, both because wall stress eventually increases and because of an intrinsic loss of contractility.[9] The mechanisms causing contractile dysfunction are under investigation but include abnormal calcium handling and exercise-induced ischemia.[10,11] The presence of diastolic and systolic dysfunction causes the symptoms of dyspnea and other symptoms of heart failure. The pathophysiology of syncope is less certain but often attributed to reduced cardiac output and decreasing peripheral resistance during exercise in the presence of reduced LV cavity size,[12] or to a vasodepressor response caused by exercise-induced obliteration of the hypertrophied LV cavity.[13]

Physical Examination

The diagnosis of AS may first be suspected when the typically harsh systolic ejection murmur is detected during physical examination. This murmur is often described as a crescendo-decrescendo murmur, but, as stenosis worsens, the murmur peaks progressively later in systole until it is primarily a crescendo murmur that radiates to

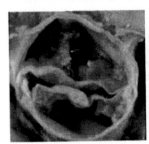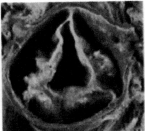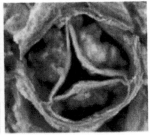

Fig. 1. Pathology specimens of stenotic aortic valves. From left: a bicuspid valve, a rheumatic valve, and a tricuspid valve. (*From* Sorajja P, Nishimura R. Aortic stenosis. In: Wang A, Bashore TM, editors. Valvular heart disease. New York: Humana Press; 2009; with permission.)

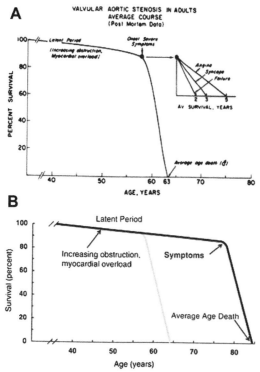

Fig. 2. The natural history of AS, as published in 1968[4] (*A*), modified by changes in cause (*B*).[3] The change from mostly rheumatic AS to atherosclerotic calcific AS causes symptom onset to occur later in life but in both cases prognosis worsens dramatically at symptom onset. (*From* Ross J Jr, Braunwald E. Aortic stenosis. Circulation 1968;38 (Suppl 1):61–7; with permission.)

the neck. In many cases the murmur is loudest in the aortic area, diminishes over the sternum, reappearing toward the LV apex (Gallavardin phenomenon), misleading the examiner into believing that a second murmur of MR is present. The carotid upstrokes are decreased in volume and delayed in the time to reach their peak (parvus et tardus). When examiners palpate the powerful sustained apical impulse of the hypertrophied LV, simultaneously with the weakened delayed carotid upstroke, they can surmise that there is an obstruction to flow between the LV and its outflow to the neck and that there is severe AS. In addition to these findings, the aortic component of the second heart sound is often lost because the valve neither opens nor closes well, so that only the pulmonic component is heard, producing a soft single second sound.

DIAGNOSTIC TESTS

Diagnostic tests in AS are designed to confirm the diagnosis suggested from physical examination, establishing disease severity and adding objectivity to the subjective nature of the history of symptoms.

Echocardiography

In all VHDs echocardiography is the mainstay of diagnosis; AS is no exception. The test establishes valve morphology, valve mobility, LV function, and the degree of LVH. Doppler interrogation of the valve establishes the velocity of flow across the valve. Flow (F) = velocity (V) × area (A). As the blood stream exiting the LV reaches the reduced area of the stenotic aortic valve, velocity must increase for flow to remain constant. Thus F_1 (ventricular flow) = F_2 (aortic flow) so that $A_1 \times V_1 = A_2 \times V_2$ and $A_2 = A_1 \times V_1/V_2$. Using a modified Bernoulli equation transvalvular gradient (g) = $4v^2$ (**Fig. 3**).[14] AS is considered severe when aortic valve area (AVA) is less than 1.0 cm², or jet velocity greater than 4 m/s, or mean transvalvular gradient greater than 40 mm Hg.[15] The criteria listed earlier may not apply when flow is reduced because of ventricular dysfunction. Three-dimensional echocardiography, which uses a matrix array transducer, can be used to planimeter the valve en fosse, establishing an anatomic valve area. However, because fluid moving through an orifice tends to stream through its center, anatomic valve area exceeds physiologic valve area and it is the latter to which the definition of severity pertains. Most importantly, no single parameter should be used to judge AS severity; all data, including the history and physical examination, valve motion, and echo-Doppler data, are used in the final analysis of valve severity. Because congenital bicuspid aortic valve is common and also is frequently associated with aortic root disorder leading to aortic dilatation and the possible need for root replacement, aortic root dimensions are assessed at the time of echocardiography.

Other Imaging Modalities

Although echocardiography remains the imaging modality of choice, cardiac MRI and computed tomography (CT) angiography fulfill specific niches in the evaluation of patients with AS. MRI can assess blood velocity and gradient in patients with poor sonographic windows not amenable to echocardiography. CT angiography is especially suited for defining both peripheral vascular anatomy and aortic annular dimensions in preparation for transcatheter valve replacement (discussed later).

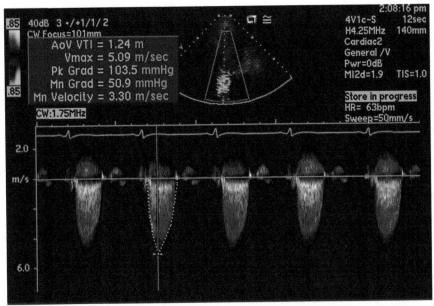

Fig. 3. The Doppler examination of a stenotic aortic valve. The jet velocity is 4 m/s. Using the modified Bernoulli equation, peak gradient = 4 (4)² = 64 mm Hg.

Stress Testing

Because some patients may not recognize their symptoms or may deny them, a formal treadmill exercise test may reveal latent symptoms and/or hemodynamic abnormalities, such as failure for blood pressure to increase with exercise. Although contraindicated in symptomatic patients, this test may be helpful in risk stratifying asymptomatic patients in whom a positive test is considered by many to be an indication for aortic valve replacement (AVR).[15–17]

Natriuretic Peptides

The pressure overload of AS may require increased preload to maintain cardiac output, in turn causing an increase in natriuretic peptides, especially B (brain)-type natriuretic peptide (BNP), which may presage decompensation. Although no value of BNP is agreed on as mandating AVR, increasing BNP on sequential follow-up examinations is worrisome and may help to steer management toward AVR.[18–21]

Cardiac Catheterization

In most cases, echocardiography provides all the data needed for complete evaluation. However, occasionally the severity of AS remains unclear after noninvasive evaluation. Cardiac catheterization provides direct measurement of the transvalvular pressure gradient and cardiac output, allowing calculation of the valve area using the Gorlin formula, in which AVA = CO/44.3 $\sqrt{g}$, with CO being cardiac output.

Therapy

AS is a mechanical obstruction to LV outflow. There is no effective medical therapy for the disease. In contrast, AVR has a remarkable benefit by dramatically improving both longevity and life span in symptomatic patients (**Fig. 4**).[22] Standard therapy is surgical

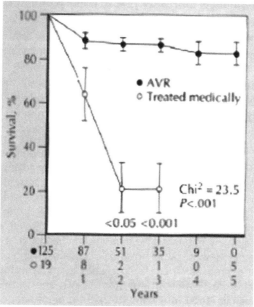

Fig. 4. The dramatic survival benefit for patients with severe AS undergoing AVR compared with patients who refused surgery. (*Adapted from* Schwarz F, Baumann P, Manthey J, et al. The effect of aortic valve replacement on survival. Circulation 1982;66:1107; with permission.)

replacement with a substitute valve. However, in high-risk patients, the transcatheter AVR (TAVR) technique permits AVR without open heart surgery.[23,24] TAVR is performed by inserting a collapsed valve, usually through the femoral artery, and advancing it to the aortic annulus where the valve is expanded, pushing aside the native valve and relieving the outflow obstruction, enhancing lifestyle and longevity.[23,24]

Special Cases

Asymptomatic patients with severe aortic stenosis

As noted earlier, the risk of sudden death in asymptomatic patients is generally less than 1%/y. However, some asymptomatic patients are at higher risk, including patients with very severe AS and a jet velocity greater than 5 m/s,[25] patients with an abnormal exercise tolerance test,[16,17] and patients with severe disease in whom serial studies have shown very rapid progression (AVA decreasing by 0.3 cm^2/y).[26]

Patient with low flow and low gradient

The standard definitions for AS severity are based on the assumption of a normal stroke volume because stroke volume generates transvalvular velocity and gradient. However, some patients have reduced stroke volume wherein transvalvular velocity and gradient are reduced but AS is severe. In some cases reduced stroke volume occurs from severe systolic dysfunction from far-advanced disease.[27] Risk of surgery is increased in such patients but is mitigated in patients who show improved LV performance with infusion of dobutamine (positive inotropic reserve).[28] In other patients, reduced stroke volume accrues from extensive LVH that restricts LV volume. Such patients still benefit from AVR if they are symptomatic and AVA and valve appearance at imaging are all consistent with severe AS.[29]

AORTIC REGURGITATION
Chronic Aortic Regurgitation

Relationship of pathophysiology to symptoms

Aortic regurgitation (AR) occurs when a disorder of either the aortic root or of the valve leaflets causes failure of leaflet coaptation. Common causes of root disorder leading to AR include Marfan syndrome, the aortopathy associated with bicuspid valve, ankylosing spondylitis, and aortic dissection. Common leaflet disorders causing AR include infective endocarditis, rheumatic valvulitis, bicuspid valve, and trauma. Formerly classified as a volume overload lesion, it is clear that AR subjects the LV to a combined pressure and volume overload.[30] The volume leaked into the LV during diastole requires the LV to increase total stroke volume to compensate for volume lost to regurgitation. However, the increased total stroke volume increases pulse pressure and accordingly increases systolic blood pressure. Increased systolic pressure in combination with a large LV radius increases systolic wall stress (afterload). Afterload in AR can be nearly as high as is seen in AS, the classic pressure overload. Concomitant development of both eccentric and concentric hypertrophy[31] can allow normal forward output at fairly normal filling pressures, so the patients with severe AR can be well compensated and asymptomatic for many years. However, eventually compensation fails, afterload increases, LV compliance decreases, filling pressures increase, and forward output decreases. These changes cause the symptoms of dyspnea on exertion, which is the most common symptom of AR. The wide pulse pressure of AR may reduce diastolic aortic pressure so that it cannot support coronary blood flow, causing angina in patients with normal epicardial coronary arteries. Reduced diastolic blood pressure may also cause syncope. As with AS (and all VHD), the onset of symptoms worsens prognosis and is an indication for AVR (**Fig. 5**).[32] Other

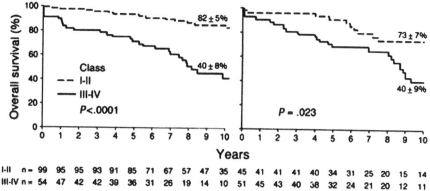

Fig. 5. The impact of preoperative symptoms on outcomes of patients with AR is dramatic both when systolic function is preserved (*left panel*) or impaired (*right panel*). (*Adapted from* Klodas E, Enriquez-Sarano M, Tajik AJ, et al. Optimizing timing of surgical correction in patients with severe aortic regurgitation: role of symptoms. J Am Coll Cardiol 1997;30:749; with permission.)

symptoms of AR include flushing during exercise, an unpleasant awareness of the heart beat, and carotid pain.

Physical examination

The physical examination of patients with severe AR is among the most impressive in cardiology. The large total stroke volume and consequent wide pulse pressure create a myriad of signs aiding in the diagnosis. The apical impulse is displaced downward and to the left and is often easily visible. The typical murmur is a diastolic blowing sound heard best along the left sternal boarder with the patient sitting up and leaning forward. Impingement of the regurgitant jet on the mitral valve causes it to vibrate and partially close during diastole, producing a diastolic rumble akin to that of mitral stenosis (Austin-Flint murmur). The carotid pulse has a bounding quality with a sharp upstroke and rapid descent (Corrigan pulse). The large stroke volume can cause head bobbing (de Musset sign). Traction on the fingernail may produce systolic plethora and diastolic blanching of the nail bed (Quincke pulse), whereas compression of the femoral artery with the bell of the stethoscope causes a to-and-fro murmur (Duroziez sign). Distortion of the pulse wave as it travels distally may cause systolic pressure in the leg to exceed that of the arm by greater than 40 mm Hg (Hill sign).

Diagnostic tests

The electrocardiogram (ECG) often shows evidence of LVH and the chest radiograph usually shows cardiac enlargement. However, the most effective diagnostic test is echocardiography, which that assesses the pathoanatomy responsible for the AR, AR severity, and its effect on chamber size and function. It also assess aortic root diameter, which is increased in some causes of AR and may lead to root replacement at the time of AVR.

Therapy

Medical therapy Several small trials of a variety of drugs, including angiotensin-converting enzyme inhibitors, angiotensin receptor blockers, and β-blockers, have examined their ability to forestall progression of the disease and the need for surgery. None have been conclusive.[33-35] For patients who have already developed heart failure, treatment with guideline-driven therapy is appropriate. However, there is also the unproven worry that β-blockers, which slow heart rate and increase the length of diastole, might also worsen AR severity.

Aortic valve replacement Aortic valve replacement (or in some cases aortic valve repair) is the only effective therapy for severe AR. By timing AVR properly, prognosis is enhanced. Thus AVR should occur when symptoms develop[32] or when asymptomatic LV dysfunction is developing as indicated by an EF decreasing toward 0.50 or when end systolic dimension approaches 50 to 55 mm.[15,32,36] As noted earlier, some patients with bicuspid aortic valve and AR also have an aortopathy with a depletion of medial elastic fibers causing dilatation of the aortic root. When root or ascending aorta diameter approaches 55 mm (or 45 mm in Marfan syndrome) the risk of aortic dissection increases and surgery to replace the aortic root at the time of AVR should be undertaken,[15] especially if there is a family history of aortic dissection.

ACUTE AORTIC REGURGITATION

Severe acute AR as might occur from leaflet perforation caused by infective endocarditis is usually a rapidly fatal illness unless recognized and treated with AVR.[37,38] However, unlike in chronic AR, which produces a dynamic, impressive physical examination, acute AR may be difficult to recognize. The LV enlargement that increases the total stroke volume and widened pulse pressure responsible for many of the signs of chronic AR has not yet developed, thus those signs are absent. Because the leaking valve results in a rapid decline of diastolic aortic pressure and rapid filling of the LV causes a steep increase in LV pressure, the pressure gradient driving AR is only present in early diastole so that the murmur is soft and unimpressive. Rapid LV filling causes LV pressure to exceed left atrial (LA) pressure before LV systole, thus closing the mitral valve prematurely. Accordingly S_1 is only composed of tricuspid valve closing and is soft. Signs of heart failure may also be subtle, marked only by an increasing pulse rate and orthopnea. When acute AR is suspected and infective endocarditis is the suspected cause, blood cultures and an echocardiogram are obtained immediately. The combination of confirmed severe acute AR with any element of clinical heart failure or echocardiographic evidence of mitral valve preclosure is an indication for emergent AVR. Although reinfection of the prosthetic replacement valve is a concern, its occurrence is rare; less than 5% even within 48 hours of obtaining a positive blood culture. Thus worry about reinfection should not be the cause of undue delay in performing lifesaving AVR.[39,40]

MITRAL STENOSIS

The most common cause of mitral stenosis (MS) is rheumatic heart disease, accounting for about 90% of cases. Although rheumatic fever is rare in developed nations, it remains common in the developing world. The attack rate for rheumatic fever is roughly equal among the sexes but MS is a disease of women, occurring about 3 times more frequently in women than in men. Patients often become aware of the disease during pregnancy when the 70% increase in cardiac output demand during the second trimester increases transvalvular gradient, causing symptom onset. Occasionally, and especially in older patients, nonrheumatic calcification of the mitral annulus also can cause significant narrowing of the mitral orifice.

Relationship of Pathophysiology to Symptoms

In normal subjects there is rapid equalization of LA and LV pressure during diastole as the open 4.0-cm mitral orifice forms a nearly common LA-LV chamber. However, as the rheumatic process compromises mitral orifice area, a pressure gradient between and LA and LV develops (**Fig. 6**),[41] increasing LA pressure, while simultaneously limiting LV filling and cardiac output. Increased LA pressure causes the symptoms of pulmonary congestion (ie, dyspnea on exertion, orthopnea, and paroxysmal nocturnal dyspnea [PND]). Thus the symptoms of left heart failure occur despite what is usually normal LV myocardial function. However, in some cases, especially in developing countries where the rheumatic process is often very aggressive, there may also be myocardial damage and LV dysfunction.[42] Because it is the RV that ultimately provides the force driving blood across the mitral valve, increased RV pressure overload (pulmonary hypertension) ensues. As MS worsens, secondary pulmonary vasoconstriction augments pulmonary pressure and severe RV pressure overload causes right-sided heart failure and the symptoms of edema and ascites. Hemoptysis is a common symptom of MS, and is not seen in other heart diseases. It occurs as the sudden increase in LA pressure during exercise ruptures thin pulmonary vein anastomoses.

Physical Examination

The pressure driving blood across the stenotic mitral valve is low (compared with AS), thus the physical findings may be subtle, and examination should occur in a quiet room and be done partially in the left lateral decubitus position. Because the transmitral gradient holds the valve open for the duration of diastole, the valve closes from its full-open (although narrowed) position, causing S_1 to be loud in most cases. However, in very severe disease the valve motion is so compromised that S_1 may be diminished. S_2 is physiologically split but its P_2 component may be loud if pulmonary hypertension has intervened. S_2 is followed by an opening snap (OS), providing a guide to disease

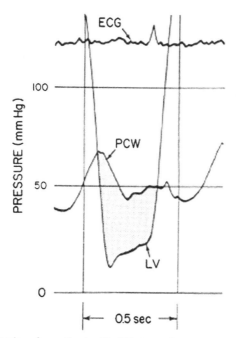

Fig. 6. The hemodynamics of a patient with MS show the LA-LV pressure gradient. PCW, pulmonary capillary wedge. (*From* Carabello BA, Grossman W. Calculation of stenotic valve orifice area. In: Baim D, Grossman W, editors. Cardiac catheterization, angiography and intervention. 5th edition. Baltimore (MD): Williams & Wilkins; 1996. p. 155; with permission.)

severity. As MS worsens, LA pressure increases, so LV and LA pressure equalize early in diastole, causing the S_2-OS interval to be short (<80 milliseconds). Lower LA pressure in milder disease leads to a longer S_2-OS interval. As rough guides, the normal splitting of the 2 components of S_2 during inspiration is 40 milliseconds, whereas the familiar cadence of S_2-S_3 is about 140 milliseconds, giving the examiner points of reference for estimating S_2-OS. Because rapid filling of the LV is nearly prohibited by MS, S_3 and S_4 are almost never heard. Following the OS, the typical diastolic low-pitched rumble of MS commences. It is best heard at the apex with the patient in the left lateral decubitus position. If the patient is in sinus rhythm, atrial contraction causes presystolic accentuation of the murmur. If pulmonary hypertension has developed, an RV lift, loud P_2, elevated neck veins, edema, and ascites may be present.

Diagnostic Tests

Atrial fibrillation is common in MS and is more related to aging than to LA size. The arrhythmia should be documented by ECG. The classic findings on chest radiograph include an enlarged pulmonary artery; a double density at the right heart border, reflecting the enlarged LA as it protrudes behind the right atrium; and Kerley B lines, the hypertrophied and scarred septa between lung lobes caused by constantly increased LA pressure. However, the definitive diagnostic modality is echocardiography **(Fig. 7)**, a test that images the mitral valve especially well. The valve area can be gauged by several techniques and valve anatomy is assessed with respect to its suitability for balloon mitral valvotomy (BMV). If even mild tricuspid regurgitation is present, the tricuspid pressure gradient can be used to calculate RV and pulmonary artery peak systolic pressure using the modified Bernoulli equation (discussed earlier). A mitral valve area of less than 1.5 cm^2 and/or a transmitral gradient greater than 5 mm Hg indicate severe MS. When symptoms and MS severity seem discordant, cardiac catheterization to assess intracardiac pressures and cardiac output at rest and during exercise often clarifies the diagnosis. In many cases normal pressures at rest become markedly increased during even mild exercise, helping to explain the patient's symptoms and suggesting that valve intervention is indicated.

Therapy

For patients with MS in atrial fibrillation the risk of stroke approaches 15%/y. Thus anticoagulation with a vitamin K antagonist is mandatory unless the risk of bleeding is severe. Control of heart rate with calcium channel blockers, β-blockers, and/or digoxin is key to permitting enough diastolic filling time for the left atrium to empty, thus

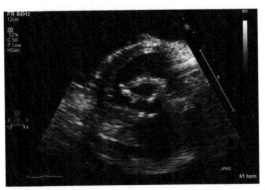

Fig. 7. An en fosse short-axis echocardiographic view or the narrowed mitral orifice from a patient with MS showing the fish-mouth appearance typical of the disease.

reducing LA pressure while maintaining cardiac output. Ultimately this mechanical obstruction to LV inflow requires a mechanical solution. In most cases this is provided by BMV, wherein a large balloon is introduced percutaneously from the right femoral vein into the right atrium. Transseptal puncture allows passage into the LA, from where the balloon is advanced to the mitral valve and inflated, mobilizing the commissural adhesions responsible for the narrowed orifice (**Fig. 8**).[43–47] BMV in most cases provides dramatic and durable relief from MS and is indicated if symptoms have developed.[45–47] Suitability for BMV is determined by valve anatomy using a scoring system that evaluates leaflet mobility, calcification, thickness, and subvalvular involvement.[48] More than mild MR is a contraindication to the procedure because it may cause the MR to worsen. If BMV is not judged to be feasible, surgical mitral valve replacement is undertaken.

PRIMARY MITRAL REGURGITATION

The mitral valve is a complex structure composed of its annulus, its leaflets, the chordae tendineae, and the papillary muscles that secure the chordae to the endocardium. Primary MR occurs when one or more of these components fails, allowing systolic retrograde flow into the LA. The most common cause of MR in the United States is myxomatous degeneration of the valve (also called mitral valve prolapse or Barlow valve). In its simplest form there may be a single chordal rupture allowing part of a leaflet to flail into the LA. In its most complex form there may be extraordinary redundancy of leaflet tissue preventing

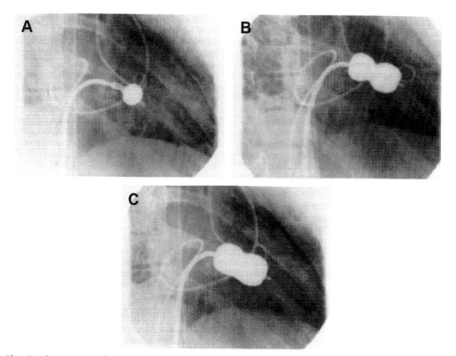

Fig. 8. The stages of Inoue BMV. (*A*) Inflation of distal balloon anchors the device against the ventricular side of the mitral valve. (*B*) Inflation of both portions of the balloon showing the waist where the balloon is indented by the stenotic valve. (*C*) Final inflation with disappearance of the waist. (*From* Iung B, Vahanian A. Rheumatic mitral valve disease. In: Otto C, Bonow R, editors. Valvular heart disease. 4th edition. Philadelphia: Elsevier; 2014. p. 264; with permission.)

a tight seal during systole (**Fig. 9**).[49] Other causes include infective endocarditis, rheumatic heart disease, and connective tissue disorders such as Marfan syndrome.

Relationship of Pathophysiology to Symptoms

In acute MR (AMR), as might occur with a chordal rupture, the small LA suddenly receives a large systolic volume of blood, greatly increasing LA pressure.[50] Simultaneously, cardiac output decreases, resulting in acute decompensation, pulmonary edema, and a low output state or even shock (**Fig. 10**). However, if MR develops more gradually, the LV and LA enlarge, allowing total stroke volume to increase, compensating the volume lost to regurgitation. In concert, the enlarged chambers can accommodate the increased volumes at lower or even normal filling pressure. As such, patients with severe MR may be asymptomatic even during exercise. However, uncorrected severe MR is not tolerated indefinitely. Persistent volume overload eventually causes LV damage, leading to the typical symptoms of heart failure (ie, dyspnea, orthopnea PND ascites, and edema). If untreated, death ensues.

Physical Examination

In AMR, the rapid equalization of systolic LA and LV pressures produces a soft, short systolic murmur that is understated compared with the patient's serious condition and

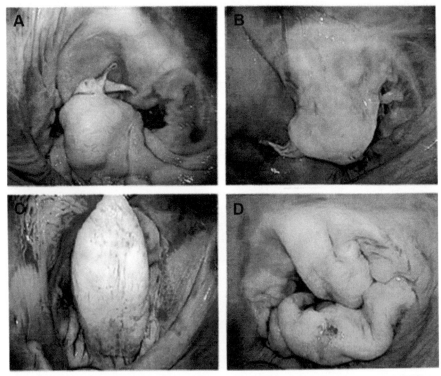

Fig. 9. The progressive pathoanatomy of myxomatous mitral valve degeneration. (*A*) Fibroelastic deficiency disease (FED) with a simple ruptured chord. (*B*) FED with multiple ruptured chords. (*C*) Barlow valve with a flail leaflet. (*D*) Extensive degeneration of both leaflets. (*From* Adams DH, Carabello BA, Castillo JG. Mitral valve regurgitation. In: Fuster V, Walsh RA, Harrington RA, editors. Hurst's the heart. 13th edition. New York: McGraw Hill; 2011. p. 1724; with permission.)

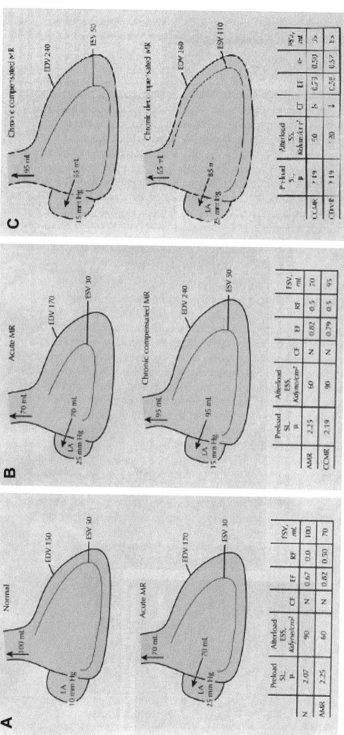

Fig. 10. The stages of MR. (A) Normal physiology compared with that of AMR. In AMR, end diastolic volume (EDV) increases slightly as preload reserve (sarcomere length [SL]) is maximized. Afterload (end systolic stress [ESS]) is reduced, facilitating ejection so that end systolic volume (ESV) is reduced. These changes act in concert with normal contractile function (CF) to increase total stroke volume, but because MR produces a regurgitant fraction (RF) of 0.5, forward stroke volume (FSV) is reduced. The excess volume displaced into the LA during systole increases LA pressure. Thus, despite normal CF, the elements of heart failure are present. (B) AMR compared with chronic compensated MR (CCMR). Eccentric hypertrophy has greatly increased EDV, whereas a return to normal afterload has increased ESV slightly. The result is a large increase in FSV. At the same time, an enlarged LA now can accommodate the regurgitant volume at nearly normal filling pressure. Despite severe MR, the elements of heart failure have been compensated. (C) CCMR compared with chronic decompensated MR (CDMR). Reduced CF and increased afterload cause a large increase in ESV, decreasing total and FSVs. LA pressure is again increased, reflecting the increased filling pressure of a failing LV. Despite the reduction in CF, increased preload maintains EF in the normal range. (Adapted from Carabello BA. Mitral regurgitation: basic pathophysiologic principles. Mod Concepts Cardiovasc Dis 1988;57:56; with permission.)

can easily be overlooked. In chronic MR the apical beat is displaced downward and to the left. S_1 is usually soft, followed by a loud holosystolic apical murmur, often radiating toward the axilla. It may be followed by S_3, indicating severe volume overload but not necessarily heart failure.

Diagnostic Tests

Echocardiography is by far the most important diagnostic test and virtually mandatory to define any case of MR. Transthoracic echo (**Fig. 11**) is usually adequate to assess the anatomic abnormalities causing the MR, MR severity, LA and LV chamber size and function, and pulmonary artery pressure when any tricuspid regurgitation is present. If transthoracic images are of nondiagnostic quality, transesophageal echocardiography provides exceptionally clear images of the valve, LA, and LV. Lesion severity is ascertained using an integrative approach that includes findings from the physical examination and qualitative and quantitative echocardiographic parameters. Factors indicating severe MR include a large color jet, an effective regurgitant orifice area greater than 0.4 cm^2, a regurgitant fraction of 0.5, a regurgitant flow of 60 mL/beat, and/or systolic pulmonary vein flow reversal.[15]

Therapy

In AMR, potent vasodilators such as sodium nitroprusside may be used to lower arterial resistance, enhancing forward flow while simultaneously decreasing regurgitant flow and LA pressure. If hypotension has intervened, vasodilators that reduce blood pressure are deleterious and intra-aortic balloon counterpulsation is used to enhance forward flow while reducing MR.[51] After stabilization, mitral surgery is used to repair the valve. In chronic MR the only effective therapy is mechanical restoration of mitral valve competence. Because the mitral valve is not just a valve but is also an integral part of the LV, aiding in LV contraction and maintaining LV shape, mitral repair is strongly preferred to replacement for restoring mitral competence.[15,52–55] Repair has approximately one-half the operative mortality of replacement and leads to better long-term symptom-free survival.[53] For rheumatic valves that may be impossible to repair, chordal sparing replacement is preferred, wherein the native connections of the leaflets to the papillary muscles are retained, aiding LV contraction. To help prevent irreversible LV dysfunction that would lead to a poor postoperative outcome, mitral repair should be performed when even mild symptoms occur.[56] Repair is performed in asymptomatic patients who develop LV dysfunction indicated by LV EF decreasing toward 0.60[57] (EF is normally 0.7 in

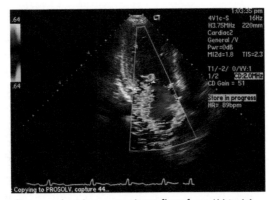

Fig. 11. An echocardiogram showing regurgitant flow from LV to LA.

MR because of favorable loading conditions that enhance ejection) or when LV end-systolic dimension approaches 40 mm.[58] If echocardiography indicates anatomy favorable to repair, many clinicians elect to correct severe MR before the benchmarks discussed earlier are reached because progression to these triggers for surgery occurs rapidly, at the rate of 8%/y.[59] In patients too ill to undergo surgery, a percutaneous approach using a clip (MitraClip, Abbott Park, North Chicago, IL) that reduces MR by joining the leaflets at their midpoints can be used.[60]

SECONDARY MITRAL REGURGITATION

Secondary (also known as functional) MR occurs when LV dysfunction, wall motion abnormalities, and dilatation prevent a normal mitral valve from coapting. It is a disease virtually separate from primary MR because the problem is severe LV disease accruing from myocardial infarction or from cardiomyopathy that has led to MR. As such, correcting the MR cannot be expected to correct the major ventricular dysfunction that caused the MR. Thus secondary MR has a different prognosis and therapy from that of primary MR.

Relationship of Pathophysiology to Symptoms

Virtually all patients with secondary MR have heart failure and the symptoms of dyspnea, orthopnea, PND, and edema that accompany it. Thus it is often difficult, if not impossible, to judge the symptoms are caused by heart failure versus those that might be being contributed to by MR.

Physical Examination

The physical examination for secondary MR is similar to that of primary MR with the exceptions that signs of heart failure are usually present and that the murmur is often softer because the LV generates less force to cause it.

Diagnostic Tests

An ECG is obtained in every case to look for evidence of previous myocardial infarction. Conduction delay may indicate that cardiac resynchronization therapy (CRT) may be useful in treating the heart failure as well in reducing MR severity. As with all other valve diseases, echocardiography is the mainstay of diagnosis. It confirms that the mitral valve is normal, establishes the severity of MR, establishes the mechanism of malcoaptation, and examines the extent of LV dysfunction. A variety of tests, including nuclear imaging and cardiac MRI, can be used to examine for myocardial viability in cases of ischemic cardiomyopathy. Large areas of myocardial viability when revascularized may lead to improved LV function and reduced MR.

Therapy

Standard guideline-directed therapy for heart failure is used in almost all cases and CRT should be considered when conduction abnormalities suggest that it may be successful. Mechanical correction of MR is considered only when the patient remains very symptomatic after standard medical therapy. This large departure from therapy for primary MR stems from there being no evidence that mechanical therapy for secondary MR prolongs life.[61–64] Also unlike in primary MR, in which mitral valve repair is highly preferred to valve replacement, there is no convincing evidence of repair superiority in secondary MR.[65,66]

SUMMARY

Each valve lesion produces a unique set of loading conditions and pathophysiology leading to a unique physical examination and unique effects on the LV and RV. However, some important generalizations can be made (with the exception of secondary MR, which is a ventricular as opposed to a valvular disease):

1. Symptom onset represents a negative demarcation in the natural history of every VHD, requiring action by the practitioner.
2. Echocardiography is the mainstay of clinical diagnosis.
3. All severe VHD is eventually fatal if left untreated.
4. All VHDs are mechanical problems that have only mechanical solutions for definitive therapy.
5. When practiced well, therapy restores lifespan to, or toward, normal.

REFERENCES

1. Otto CM, Kuusisto J, Reichenbach DD, et al. Characterization of the early lesion of 'degenerative' valvular aortic stenosis: histological and immunohistochemical studies. Circulation 1994;90:844–53.
2. Sorajja P, Nishimura R. Aortic stenosis. In: Wang A, Bashore TM, editors. Valvular heart disease. London: Human Press; 2009. p. 167.
3. Carabello BA. Introduction to aortic stenosis. Circ Res 2013;113(2):179–85.
4. Ross J Jr, Braunwald E. Aortic stenosis. Circulation 1968;38(Suppl 1):61–7.
5. Marcus ML, Doty DB, Hiratzka LF, et al. Decreased coronary reserve: a mechanism for angina pectoris in patients with aortic stenosis and normal coronary arteries. N Engl J Med 1982;307:1362–6.
6. Rajappan K, Rimoldi OE, Camici PG, et al. Functional changes in coronary microcirculation after valve replacement in patients with aortic stenosis. Circulation 2003;107:3170–5.
7. Zile MR, Brutsaert DL. New concepts in diastolic dysfunction and diastolic heart failure: part II, casual mechanisms and treatment. Circulation 2002;105:1503–8.
8. Hess OM, Ritter M, Schneider J, et al. Diastolic stiffness and myocardial structural I aortic valve disease before and after valve replacement. Circulation 1984;69: 855–65.
9. Huber D, Grimm J, Koch R, et al. Determinants of ejection performance in aortic stenosis. Circulation 1981;64:126–34.
10. Nakano K, Corin WJ, Spann JF Jr, et al. Abnormal subendocardial blood flow in pressure overload hypertrophy is associated with pacing-induced subendocardial dysfunction. Circ Res 1989;65:1555–64.
11. Ho K, Yan X, Feng X, et al. Transgenic expression of sarcoplasmic reticulum Ca(2+) ATPase modifies the transition from hypertrophy to early heart failure. Circ Res 2001;89:422–9.
12. Park SJ, Enriquez-Sarano M, Chang SA, et al. Hemodynamic patterns for symptomatic presentations of severe aortic stenosis. JACC Cardiovasc Imaging 2013; 6:137–46.
13. Mark AL, Abboud FM, Schmid PG, et al. Reflex vascular responses of left ventricular outflow obstruction and activation of ventricular baroreceptors I dogs. J Clin Invest 1973;52(5):1147–53.
14. Otto CM, Pearlman AS, Comess KA, et al. Determination of the stenotic aortic valve area in adults using Doppler echocardiography. J Am Coll Cardiol 1986; 7:509–17.

15. Nishimura RA, Otto CM, Bonow RO, et al, American College of Cardiology/American Heart Association Task Force on Practice Guidelines. 2014 AHA/ACC guideline for the management of patients with valvular heart disease: a report of the American College of Cardiology/American Heart Association Task Force on Practice Guidelines. J Am Coll Cardiol 2014;63(22):e57–185.
16. Das P, Rimington H, Chambers J. Exercise testing to stratify risk in aortic stenosis. Eur Heart J 2005;26:1309–13.
17. Amato MC, Moffa PJ, Werner KE, et al. Treatment decision in asymptomatic aortic valve stenosis: role of exercise testing. Heart 2001;86:381–6.
18. Gerber IL, Legget ME, West TM, et al. Usefulness of serial measurement of N-terminal pro-brain natriuretic peptide plasma levels in asymptomatic patients with aortic stenosis to predict symptomatic deterioration. Am J Cardiol 2005;95: 898–901.
19. Bergler-Klein J, Klaar U, Heger M, et al. Natriuretic peptides predict symptom-free survival and postoperative outcome in severe aortic stenosis. Circulation 2004;109:2302–8.
20. Nessmith MG, Fukuta H, Brucks S, et al. Usefulness of an elevated B-type natriuretic peptide in predicting survival I patients with aortic stenosis treated without surgery. Am J Cardiol 2005;96:1445–8.
21. Steadman CD, Ray S, Ng LL, et al. Natriuretic peptides in common valvular heart disease. J Am Coll Cardiol 2010;55:2034–48.
22. Schwarz F, Baumann P, Manthey J, et al. The effect of aortic valve replacement on survival. Circulation 1982;66:1105–10.
23. Kodali SK, Williams MR, Smith CR, et al, PARTNER Trial Investigators. Two-year outcomes after transcatheter or surgical aortic-valve replacement. N Engl J Med 2012;366(18):1686–95.
24. Adams DH, Popma JJ, Reardon MJ, et al, U.S. CoreValve Clinical Investigators. Transcatheter aortic-valve replacement with a self-expanding prosthesis. N Engl J Med 2014;370(19):1790–8.
25. Rosenhek R, Zilberszac R, Schemper M, et al. Natural history of very severe aortic stenosis. Circulation 2010;121:151–6.
26. Rosenhek R, Binder T, Porenta G, et al. Predictors of outcome in severe asymptomatic aortic stenosis. N Engl J Med 2000;343:611–7.
27. Carabello BA, Green LH, Grossman W, et al. Hemodynamic determinants of prognosis of aortic valve replacement in critical aortic stenosis and advanced congestive heart failure. Circulation 1980;62:42–8.
28. Monin JL, Quere JP, Monchi M, et al. Low-gradient aortic stenosis: operative risk stratification and predictors for long-term outcome-a multicenter study using dobutamine stress hemodynamics. Circulation 2003;108:319–24.
29. Clavel MA, Dumesnil JG, Capoulade R, et al. Outcome of patients with aortic stenosis, small valve area, and low-flow, low-gradient despite preserved left ventricular ejection fraction. J Am Coll Cardiol 2012;60(14):1259–67.
30. Wisenbaugh T, Spann JF, Carabello BA. Differences in myocardial performance and load between patients with similar amounts of chronic aortic versus chronic mitral regurgitation. J Am Coll Cardiol 1984;3:916–23.
31. Feiring AJ, Rumberger JA. Ultrafast computed tomography analysis of regional radius-to-wall thickness ratios in normal and volume-overloaded human left ventricle. Circulation 1992;85(4):1423–32.
32. Klodas E, Enriquez-Sarano M, Tajik AJ, et al. Optimizing timing of surgical correction in patients with severe aortic regurgitation: role of symptoms. J Am Coll Cardiol 1997;30:746–52.

33. Scognamiglio R, Rahimtoola SH, Fasoli G, et al. Nifedipine in asymptomatic patients with severe aortic regurgitation and normal left ventricular function. N Engl J Med 1994;331(11):689–94.
34. Evangelista A, Tornos P, Sambola A, et al. Long-term vasodilator therapy in patients with severe aortic regurgitation. N Engl J Med 2005;353(13):1342–9.
35. Sampat U, Varadarjan P, Turk R, et al. Effect of beta-blocker therapy on survival in patients with severe aortic regurgitation results from a cohort of 756 patients. J Am Coll Cardiol 2009;54(5):452–7.
36. Henry WL, Bonow RO, Rosing DR, et al. Observations on the optimum time for operative intervention for aortic regurgitation. II. Serial echocardiographic evaluation of asymptomatic patients. Circulation 1980;61(3):484–92.
37. Mann T, McLaurin L, Grossman W, et al. Assessing the hemodynamic severity of acute aortic regurgitation due to infective endocarditis. N Engl J Med 1975; 293(3):108–13.
38. Sareli P, Klein HO, Schamroth CL, et al. Contribution of echocardiography and immediate surgery to the management of severe aortic regurgitation from active infective endocarditis. Am J Cardiol 1986;57(6):413–8.
39. al Jubair K, al Fagih MR, Ashmeg A, et al. Cardiac operations during active endocarditis. J Thorac Cardiovasc Surg 1992;104(2):487–90.
40. Yu VL, Fang GD, Keys TF, et al. Prosthetic valve endocarditis: superiority of surgical valve replacement versus medical therapy only. Ann Thorac Surg 1994; 58(4):1073–7.
41. Carabello BA, Grossman W. Calculation of stenotic valve orifice area. In: Baim D, Grossman W, editors. Cardiac catheterization, angiography and intervention. 5th edition. Baltimore (MD): Williams & Wilkins; 1996. p. 155.
42. Mohan JC, Khalilullah M, Arora R. Left ventricular intrinsic contractility in pure rheumatic mitral stenosis. Am J Cardiol 1989;64:240.
43. Iung B, Vahanian A. Rheumatic mitral valve disease. In: Otto C, Bonow R, editors. Valvular heart disease. 4th edition. Philadelphia: Elsevier; 2014. p. 264.
44. Roy SB, Gopinath N. Mitral stenosis. Circulation 1968;38(Suppl V):V-68.
45. Reyes VP, Raju BS, Wynne J, et al. Percutaneous balloon valvuloplasty compared with open surgical commissurotomy for mitral stenosis. N Engl J Med 1994; 331(15):961–7.
46. Ben Farhat M, Ayari M, Maatouk F, et al. Percutaneous balloon versus surgical closed and open mitral commissurotomy: seven-year follow-up results of a randomized trial. Circulation 1998;97(3):245–50.
47. Rifaie O, Abdel-Dayem MK, Ramzy A, et al. Percutaneous mitral valvotomy versus closed surgical commissurotomy. Up to 15 years of follow-up of a prospective randomized study. J Cardiol 2009;53(1):28–34.
48. Wilkins GT, Weyman AE, Abascal VM, et al. Percutaneous balloon dilation of the mitral valve: an analysis of echocardiographic variables related to outcome and the mechanism of dilation. Br Heart J 1988;60(4):299–308.
49. Adams DH, Carabello BA, Castillo JG. Mitral valve regurgitation. In: Fuster V, Walsh RA, Harrington RA, editors. Hurst's the heart. 13th edition. New York: McGraw Hill; 2011. p. 1724.
50. Carabello BA. Mitral regurgitation: basic pathophysiologic principles. Mod Concepts Cardiovasc Dis 1988;57:53–8.
51. Horstkotte D, Schulte HD, Niehues R, et al. Diagnostic and therapeutic considerations in acute, severe mitral regurgitation: experience in 42 consecutive patients entering the intensive care unit with pulmonary edema. J Heart Valve Dis 1993;2: 512–22.

52. Rozich JD, Carabello BA, Usher BW, et al. Mitral valve replacement with and without chordal preservation in patients with chronic mitral regurgitation. Mechanisms for differences in postoperative performance. Circulation 1992;86: 1718–26.
53. Enriquez-Sarano M, Schaff HV, Orszulak TA, et al. Valve repair improves the outcome of surgery for mitral regurgitation analysis. Circulation 1995;91:1022–8.
54. Horskotte D, Schulte HD, Bircks W, et al. The effect of chordal preservation on late outcome after mitral valve replacement: a randomized study. J Heart Valve Dis 1993;2:150–8.
55. David TE, Armstrong S, McCrindle BW, et al. Late outcomes of mitral valve repair for mitral regurgitation due to degenerative disease. Circulation 2013;127(14): 1485–92.
56. Gillinov AM, Mihaljevic T, Blackstone EH, et al. Should patients with severe degenerative mitral regurgitation delay surgery until symptoms develop? Ann Thorac Surg 2010;90(2):481–8.
57. Enriquez-Sarano M, Tajik AJ, Schaff HV, et al. Echocardiographic prediction of survival after surgical correction of organic mitral regurgitation. Circulation 1994;90:830–7.
58. Tribouilloy C, Grigioni F, Avierinos JF, et al. Survival implication of left ventricular end-systolic diameter in mitral regurgitation due to flail leaflets a long-term follow-up multicenter study. J Am Coll Cardiol 2009;54:1961–8.
59. Rosenhek R, Rader F, Klaar U, et al. Outcome of watchful waiting in asymptomatic severe mitral regurgitation. Circulation 2006;113(18):2238–44.
60. Feldman T, Foster E, Glower DD, et al. Percutaneous repair or surgery for mitral regurgitation. N Engl J Med 2011;364:1395–406.
61. Fattouch K, Guccione F, Sampognaro R, et al. POINT: efficacy of adding mitral valve restrictive annuloplasty to coronary artery bypass grafting in patients with moderate ischemic mitral valve regurgitation: a randomized trial. J Thorac Cardiovasc Surg 2009;138:278–85.
62. Mihaljevic T, Lam BK, Rajeswaran J, et al. Impact of mitral valve annuloplasty combined with revascularization in patients with functional ischemic mitral regurgitation. J Am Coll Cardiol 2007;49:2191–201.
63. Wu AH, Aaronson KD, Bolling SF, et al. Impact of mitral valve annuloplasty on mortality risk in patients with mitral regurgitation and left ventricular systolic dysfunction. J Am Coll Cardiol 2005;45:381–7.
64. Benedetto U, Melina G, Roscitano A, et al. Does combined mitral valve surgery improve survival when compared to revascularization alone in patients with ischemic mitral regurgitation? A meta-analysis on 2479 patients. J Cardiovasc Med (Hagerstown) 2009;10:109–14.
65. Cohn LH, Rizzo RJ, Adams DH, et al. The effect of pathophysiology on the surgical treatment of ischemic mitral regurgitation: operative and late risks of repair versus replacement. Eur J Cardiothorac Surg 1995;9:568–74.
66. Acker MA, Parides MK, Perrault LP, et al, CTSN. Mitral-valve repair versus replacement for severe ischemic mitral regurgitation. N Engl J Med 2014; 370(1):23–32.

New Oral Anticoagulants

Their Role in Stroke Prevention in High-Risk Patients with Atrial Fibrillation

Sunita J. Ferns, MD, MRCPCH (UK)[a], Gerald V. Naccarelli, MD, FHRS[b],*

KEYWORDS

- Anticoagulation • Novel oral anticoagulants • Atrial fibrillation • Factor IIa inhibitors
- Factor Xa inhibitors • Stroke

KEY POINTS

- Novel oral anticoagulants (NOACs) make up approximately 20% of new anticoagulant prescriptions.
- NOACs have advantages of fixed-dose oral dosing, rapid onset and offset, and fewer interactions with food and drugs compared with vitamin K antagonists (VKAs).
- NOACs are at least as effective as VKAs in patients with atrial fibrillation (AF) and venous thromboembolism.
- NOACs have similar, if not lower, rates of serious hemorrhagic complications.
- Common errors in NOAC use include inappropriate patient selection, inappropriate dose selection, and inappropriate monitoring.

INTRODUCTION

AF is the most common sustained arrhythmia and the leading cause of stroke in adults worldwide.[1,2] Traditionally, warfarin and other VKAs have been the mainstay treatment option for patients with increased risk of stroke. Their use is, however, limited by a narrow therapeutic index and interactions with multiple foods and other medications, requiring frequent monitoring and dose adjustments.[3] In the last 5 years, NOACs that inhibit thrombin or activated factor X (fXa) have been approved as an alternative to warfarin for stroke risk reduction in AF. Dabigatran etexilate, an oral reversible direct thrombin inhibitor, was the first of these agents. It was followed by rivaroxaban, apixaban, edoxaban, and, recently, betrixaban (phase 3 trials).[4–7] The NOACs offer several advantages over VKAs, such as rapid onset and offset of action, fewer drug interactions, and an absence of an effect of dietary vitamin K intake on drug activity (**Fig. 1**).[8–12] This article reviews the pharmacologic and evidence-based data as well

[a] Department of Pediatrics, University of North Carolina, College of Medicine, 101 Manning Drive, Chapel Hill, NC 27599, USA; [b] Penn State Hershey heart and Vascular Institute, Penn State College of Medicine, 500 University Drive, Hershey, PA 17033, USA
* Corresponding author.
E-mail address: gnaccarelli@hmc.psu.edu

Med Clin N Am 99 (2015) 759–780
http://dx.doi.org/10.1016/j.mcna.2015.02.006
0025-7125/15/$ – see front matter Crown Copyright © 2015 Published by Elsevier Inc. All rights reserved.
medical.theclinics.com

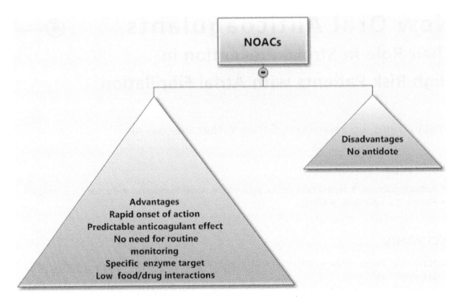

Fig. 1. Advantages and disadvantages of newer anticoagulants.

as the clinical characteristics of NOACs and their role in preventing stroke and thrombo-embolic events in high-risk patients with nonvalvular AF (NVAF). Rivaroxaban and apix-aban are also approved for the primary prevention of embolic events in patients who undergo hip and knee replacement surgery. Dabigatran, rivaroxaban, and apixaban are approved for deep vein thrombosis and pulmonary embolism (DVT/PE) treatment and prevention. Edoxaban is awaiting US Food and Drug Administration (FDA) approval.

PHARMACOLOGY

NOACs are small molecules that specifically target individual clotting factors. As thrombin is the final effector in blood coagulation, it is a logical target for newer agents. Thrombin converts fibrinogen to fibrin and also amplifies its own generation by feed-back activation of factors V, VIII, and XI. Thrombin is also a potent platelet agonist. Therefore, thrombin inhibition not only attenuates fibrin formation but also reduces thrombin generation and platelet activation. The NOACs target either thrombin or fXa (**Fig. 2**). Dabigatran etexilate is a direct thrombin inhibitor, whereas rivaroxaban, apixaban, edoxaban, and betrixaban work by direct fXa inhibition.[2,13–19] **Tables 1** and **2** detail the characteristics and drug interactions of the NOACs.[20–36]

Dabigatran Etexilate

Dabigatran etexilate, a substrate of the P-glycoprotein (P-gp) transporter, is a potent, competitive, reversible inhibitor of thrombin that acts by binding clot-bound and free thrombin with a high affinity and specificity. The prodrug, or etexilate form, is rapidly converted to dabigatran by esterases and has an oral bioavailability of 6.5%. Drug capsules are filled with tartaric acid, as drug absorption is enhanced with a low pH. Levels usually peak 2 hours after oral administration. The half-life of dabigatran is 8 hours after single dose and 14 to 17 hours after multiple doses, enabling once or twice daily administration. Dabigatran is primarily excreted by the kidneys, and there-fore caution must be exercised in patients with renal dysfunction (creatinine clearance

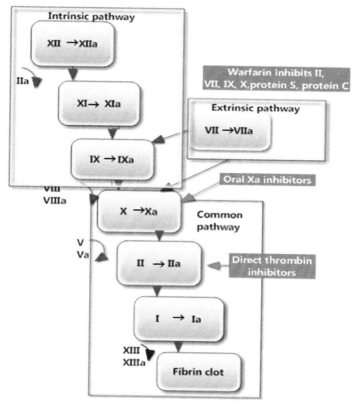

Fig. 2. Sites of action of newer anticoagulants.

[CrCl] <50 mL/min). Drug interactions are detailed in **Table 2**. Dyspepsia is the most common reported side effect (see **Table 1**).[2,8,37]

Rivaroxaban

Rivaroxaban is an active compound that acts by binding reversibly to the active site of fXa. It has an oral bioavailability of 80%, a rapid onset of action with a C_{max} of 2 to 4 hours, and a half-life of 5 to 9 hours in young individuals that increases to 11 to 13 hours in the elderly. A third of the metabolized drug is excreted by direct renal elimination and two-thirds is metabolized by the liver via cytochrome P450 (CYP) 3A4-dependent and independent pathways. Rivaroxaban is a substrate for P-gp. Administration of drugs that are strong P-gp and CYP3A4 inhibitors, such as ketoconazole or ritonavir, are contraindicated, as these increase plasma drug levels of rivaroxaban. Detailed drug interaction information are given in **Table 2**.[9,17]

Apixaban

Apixaban is a selective active site inhibitor of fXa. It does not require antithrombin III for antithrombotic activity and inhibits free and clot-bound fXa and prothrombinase activity. Although it has no direct effects on platelet aggregation, it indirectly inhibits platelet aggregation induced by thrombin. By inhibiting fXa, apixaban decreases thrombin generation and thrombus development. It is absorbed rapidly with a bioavailability of 50%, and maximal plasma concentrations are achieved in 3 to 4 hours.

Table 1
Pharmacologic features of newer anticoagulants

Drug	Dabigatran	Rivaroxaban	Apixaban	Edoxaban[a]	Betrixaban[b]
Prodrug	Yes	No	No	No	No
Factor inhibited	Thrombin	Xa	Xa	Xa	Xa
Bioavailability (%)	6	80	60	50	35
Dosing	150 mg bid 110 mg bid	20 mg daily 15 mg daily	5 mg bid 2.5 mg bid	60 mg daily 30 mg daily 15 mg daily	80 mg daily
Absorption with food	No effect	+39% more	No effect	6%–22% more	
Recommended intake with food	No	Yes	No	No	No
GI side effects	Dyspepsia	None	None	None	Nausea, diarrhea
Absorption with H2B/PPI	−12% to 30 %	None	None	None	—
Peak plasma levels (h)	2–3	2–4	1–4	1–2	3–4
Plasma trough level (h)	12–24	16–24	12–24	12–24	—
Half-life (h)	14–17	5–9	12	9–11	19–24
Renal clearance (%)	80	35	25	35	7
Liver metabolism (CYP3A4)	No	Yes	Yes	Mild	No
P-glycoprotein inhibition	Yes	Yes	Yes	Yes	Yes

Abbreviations: GI, gastrointestinal; H2B, histamine-2 blockers; PPI, proton pump inhibitors.
[a] Awaiting FDA approval.
[b] In phase 3 trials.

The half-life is 8 to 14 hours. It exhibits linear pharmacokinetics and is 87% plasma protein bound. Elimination is via multiple pathways, including hepatic metabolism via CYP3A4 and renal and intestinal excretion. It is also a substrate for P-gp transporter.[10]

Edoxaban

Edoxaban is another highly selective, competitive inhibitor of fXa. Because it is rapidly absorbed with a peak plasma concentration in 1.5 hours and a half-life of 10 to 14 hours, it may be given once daily. The bioavailability is 62%, and its activity is not influenced by food intake. The plasma concentrations of edoxaban closely correlate with suppression of thrombin generation and inhibition of a range of platelet activation parameters. One-third of the drug is eliminated via the kidney, and the remainder is excreted in the feces. Strong P-gp inhibitors, such as dronedarone, quinidine, and verapamil, require a 50% dose reduction in edoxaban. The effects of edoxaban may also be increased in patients with a body weight of 60 kg or less and moderate renal impairment.[11,12]

Betrixaban

Betrixaban is an oral once-daily fXa inhibitor. Unlike other prior agents, it has a long half-life of 15 to 20 hours and extrarenal clearance. Therefore, it can be used in

Table 2
Drug interactions of newer oral anticoagulants

Drug	Mechanism of Interference	Dabigatran	Rivaroxaban	Apixaban	Edoxaban[a]	Betrixaban[b]
Antacids	Absorption	−12% to 30%	No effect	No data	No effect	—
Antiarrhythmics						
Amiodarone	P-gp	+12% to 60%	Minor effect	No data	No effect	+260%
Dronedarone	P-gp & CYP3A4	+70% to 100%	No data	No data	+85%	—
Digoxin	P-gp	No effect	No effect	No data	No effect	No effect
Verapamil	P-gp & CYP3A4	+20% to 180%	Minor effect	No data	+53%	+450%
Diltiazem	P-gp & CYP3A4	No effect	Minor effect	+40%	No data	—
Antifungals						
Ketoconazole	CYP3A4	+140% to 150%	+160%	+100%	No data	+230%
Antiretrovirals						
HIV protease inhibitors	P-gp & CYP3A4	No data	+153%	Strong increase	No data	—
Antiepileptics						
CMZ, phenytoin, phenobarbitone	P-gp & CYP3A4	−66%	−50%	−54%	−30%	—
Miscellaneous						
Rifampicin, St. John's wort	P-gp & CYP3A4	−66%	−50%	−54%	−30%	—
Cyclosporin, tacrolimus	P-gp	No data	+50%	No data	No data	—

Abbreviations: CMZ, carbamazepine; CYP, cytochrome P450; HIV, human immunodeficiency virus.
[a] Awaiting FDA approval.
[b] In phase 3 trials.

patients with severe renal impairment. In addition, betrixaban has properties that may allow it to demonstrate efficacy without the increase in the rate of major bleeding seen with other fXa inhibitors in acute medically ill patients. It has a low peak-to-trough drug concentration ratio that minimizes anticoagulant variability. Lack of CYP3A4 metabolism reduces the risk of drug-drug interactions. Its effects can potentially be reversed with alfa (PRT4445), an investigational recombinant fXa inhibitor antidote.[38]

DRUG MONITORING WITH NOVEL ORAL ANTICOAGULANTS

The current NOACs do not require routine blood monitoring, and neither dosing nor dosage intervals should be altered in response to changes in laboratory coagulation parameters. However, testing may be performed in case of major bleeding, thrombotic events, or urgent surgery. Testing may also be required in cases of suspected overdosing, severe renal or hepatic insufficiency, or suspected drug interactions. **Table 3** lists the standard coagulation tests and their applicability in patients administered NOACs.[39–42] Unfortunately, some of these tests are not readily available in all centers.

When interpreting a test, it is essential to know when the drug was administered in relation to the blood draw, as a sample taken at peak levels demonstrates a much higher effect than one drawn at trough concentrations. With dabigatran specifically, there is a close correlation between plasma concentration and the degree of anticoagulant effect. If the blood level is 30 ng or less, one can proceed with the urgent surgery on NOACs; however, if the level is very high (eg, overdose), the risk of hemorrhage is high and dialysis should be considered before surgery. The activated partial thromboplastin time (aPTT) may also be useful to indirectly assess dabigatran activity; however, dabigatran has little or no effect on the prothrombin time (PT)

Table 3
Applicability of coagulation assays in patients administered NOACs

Drug Laboratory Test	Availability	Coagulation Phase Studied	Dabigatran	Rivaroxaban	Apixaban	Edoxaban
PT	Yes	Extrinsic/ common pathway	No	Prolonged	No	Prolonged
aPTT	Yes	Intrinsic/ common pathway	Yes (trough >2× ULN bleed)	No	No	Prolonged
INR	Yes	Extrinsic/ common pathway	No	No	No	No
dTT	Limited	DTI activity	Yes (trough >200 ng/mL-bleed)	No	No	No
ECT	Limited	DTI activity	Yes (trough >3× ULN bleed)	No	No	No
Anti-Xa activity	Limited	Specific factor	NA	Yes	Yes	Yes
Factor IIa	NA	—	Yes	No	No	—

Abbreviations: aPTT, activated partial thromboplastin time; DTI, direct thrombin inhibitor; dTT, diluted thrombin time; ECT, ecarin coagulation time; INR, International normalized ratio; PT, prothrombin time; UNL, upper limit of normal.

and international normalized ratio (INR).[39,40] The diluted thrombin time assay may be useful to indirectly assess dabigatran concentrations as it displays a direct linear relationship. The ecarin clotting time assay provides a direct measure of the activity of direct thrombin inhibitors, but both these tests are not readily available.[40–42]

For rivaroxaban the PT may provide a qualitative assessment, with a concentration-dependent prolongation of the PT noted. There are currently no such data available for edoxaban and apixaban. Anti-fXa assays are available at limited centers to assess plasma concentrations of the fXa inhibitors; however, there are no clear data showing association between drug levels and the risk of bleeding. The aPTT and INR do not provide meaningful information in the evaluation of fXa inhibitor and should not be used.[20,43]

TRIALS ON NEWER ANTICOAGULANTS

Multiple trials have been carried out to compare the use of NOACs with warfarin: RE-LY (Randomized Evaluation of Long Term Anticoagulant Therapy [RE-LY] With Dabigatran Etexilate), dabigatran; ROCKET AF (Rivaroxaban versus Warfarin in Nonvalvular Atrial Fibrillation), rivaroxaban; ARISTOTLE (Apixaban for the Prevention of Stroke in Subjects With Atrial Fibrillation), apixaban; ENGAGE TIMI-AF 48 (Global Study to Assess the Safety and Effectiveness of Edoxaban [DU-176b] vs Standard Practice of Dosing With Warfarin in Patients With Atrial Fibrillation), edoxaban; and APEX (Acute Medically Ill VTE Prevention With Extended Duration Betrixaban Study), betrixaban (phase 3 stage). Comparisons are detailed in **Table 4**. These trials did not include patients with mitral stenosis or any type of prosthetic heart valves or those likely to need a valve replacement in the near future.

Randomized Evaluation of Long Term Anticoagulant Therapy (RE-LY) With Dabigatran Etexilate

- This study compared dabigatran to warfarin in 18,113 patients with AF at risk for stroke (PROBE (Prospective, randomized, outcome blinded trial) design).
- The mean CHADS$_2$ (Diagnosed heart failure, past or current [1 point], Hypertension treated or untreated [1 point], Age $\geq$ 75 years [1 point], Diabetes Mellitus [1 point], Secondary prevention in patients with prior ischemic stroke, TIA or thromboembolism [2 points]) score was 2.1, and median follow-up duration was 2 years.
- Patients were randomly assigned to 1 of 2 blinded doses of dabigatran, 110 or 150 mg twice daily, or open-label, dose-adjusted warfarin to study primary outcome of stroke or systemic embolization.
- This condition occurred at rates of 1.71% per year in the group assigned to warfarin; 1.54% per year in those randomized to dabigatran, 110 mg twice daily ($P<.001$ for noninferiority to warfarin); and 1.11% per year with dabigatran, 150 mg twice daily ($P<.001$ for superiority to warfarin).
- Significantly lower rates of intracerebral hemorrhage were noted with both doses of dabigatran when compared with warfarin.
- The higher dose of dabigatran yielded a higher rate of gastrointestinal bleeding but a similar rate of major bleeding as compared with warfarin.
- All-cause mortality was lower with dabigatran (4.13% per year for warfarin; 3.75% per year for dabigatran, 110 mg twice daily; and 3.64% per year for dabigatran, 150 mg twice daily) but did not reach statistical significance ($P = .13$ and $P = .051$ for the 110 and 150 mg twice daily doses, respectively).[2]
- Following RE-LY, dabigatran, 150 mg twice daily, was approved to reduce the risk of stroke and systemic embolism in patients with NVAF worldwide.

Table 4
Comparison of trials studying newer anticoagulants for stroke prevention in AF

Trial	RE-LY	ROCKET-AF	ARISTOTLE	AVERROES	ENGAGE-AF	EXPLORE Xa
Drug	Dabigatran	Rivaroxaban	Apixaban	Apixaban	Edoxaban	Betrixaban
Dose	110 mg bid 150 mg bid	20 mg daily 15 mg daily[a]	5 mg bid 2.5 mg bid[a]	5 mg bid 2.5 mg bid[a]	30 mg daily 60 mg daily	40, 60, 80 mg daily
Control	Warfarin	Warfarin	Warfarin	Aspirin	Warfarin	Enoxaparin
Year	2009	2011	2011	2010	2013	2012
N	18,113	14,264	18,201	5599	21,105	561
Study design	PROBE	Double blind, double dummy, noninferiority	Double blind, double dummy, noninferiority	Double blind	Double blind, double dummy, noninferiority	Randomized blinded open label
Study population	Nonvalvular AF with >stroke risk	Nonvalvular AF with previous stroke/TIA/systemic embolism or ≥2 stroke risk factor	Nonvalvular AF with ≥1 stroke risk factor	Nonvalvular AF with ≥1 stroke risk factor, VKA unsuitable, refused, or failed	Nonvalvular AF with ≥2 stroke risk factors	Nonvalvular AF and AFl with at least 1 risk factor for stroke
AF type Persistent/ permanent: paroxysmal	2:1	4.5:1	5.67:1	2.33:1	3:1	1.18:1
Age (median) (y)	71 (mean)	73	70	70	72	74
Women (%)	37	40	36	41	39	33.5
CHADS$_2$ (mean)	2.1	3.5	2.1	2	2.8	2.2
VKA naive (%)	50	38	43	60	39	13
Prior CVA/TIA (%)	20	54.8	19.4	14	28	—
TTR (mean) (%)	64	55	62	NA	—	63.4
Median FU (y)	2	1.9	1.8	1.1	2.8	0.4
Primary efficacy end point	Stroke or STE	Stroke or STE	Stroke or STE	Stroke or STE	Stroke or STE	Time to major or clinically relevant nonmajor bleeding

Primary outcome HR	0.66	0.88	0.79	0.45	0.79	0.14, 0.7, 0.75[b]
Hem CVA rate	0.24	0.59	0.51	0.21	0.26	—
Ischemic CVA HR	0.75	0.99	0.92	0.37	1	—
Secondary efficacy end point	Ischemic, hemorrhagic, or unspecified stroke, MI, PE, hospitalization, and all-cause and vascular death	Ischemic or hemorrhagic stroke outcome, non-CNS embolism, MI, all-cause death, vascular and nonvascular death	Ischemic, hemorrhagic, unspecified stroke of unknown cause, all-cause death, MI, PE, or deep vein thrombosis		Ischemic, hemorrhagic, unspecified stroke, disabling/fatal stroke, MI, all-cause and vascular death	Stroke, systemic embolism, cardiovascular and all-cause death
Primary safety end point	Major bleeding (including life-threatening, non–life-threatening, and GI bleeding)	Major and clinically relevant nonmajor bleeding	Major bleeding (including intracranial, other organ, and GI bleeding)	Major bleeding	Major bleeding (including intracranial, extracranial, or unclassified and fatal bleeding)	Time to major or clinically relevant nonmajor bleeding
Secondary safety end point	Minor bleeding, major or minor bleeding, intracranial and extracranial bleeding, net clinical benefit	Minor bleeding (eg, epistaxis, hematuria)	Major or clinically relevant nonmajor bleeding	Clinically relevant nonmajor and minor bleeding	Major and clinically relevant nonmajor bleeding, incidence of liver enzyme/bilirubin abnormalities	Any bleeding
Major bleeding rate (%)	3.1	3.6	2.13	3.1	2.75	—
All causes death (%/y)	3.64	1.9	1.87	3.5	3.99	—

Abbreviations: AFl, atrial flutter; CNS, central nervous system; CVA, cerebrovascular accident; FU, follow-up; GI, gastrointestinal; HR, hazard ratio; MI, myocardial infarction; PE, pulmonary embolism; STE, systemic embolization; TIA, transient ischemic attack; TTR, time in treatment range.

a Select patients.
b Doses of betrixaban.

- Recently, this drug was approved by the FDA for treatment of DVT and PE.
- Although patients with severe renal impairment (CrCl <30 mL/min) were excluded from RE-LY, the FDA approved a dose of 75 mg twice daily for patients with CrCl 15 to 30 mL/min, based on pharmacokinetic modeling.

Rivaroxaban versus Warfarin in Nonvalvular Atrial Fibrillation

- This study was a double-blind, double-dummy study carried out over a median follow-up of 1.9 years comparing rivaroxaban with warfarin in 14,264 patients with NVAF who were at increased risk for stroke.[17]
- The study included patients with high stroke risk with a mean CHADS2 score of 3.5, with 55% of patients having a prior stroke or transient ischemic attack (TIA).
- Study arm patients received fixed-dose rivaroxaban, 20 mg once daily (15 mg daily for those with CrCl 30–49 mL/min).
- Rivaroxaban was superior to warfarin (hazard ratio [HR], 0.88; $P = .015$) in preventing stroke or systemic embolism.
- Rivaroxaban reduced the frequency of hemorrhagic strokes compared with warfarin by 41% (HR, 0.59).

Apixaban for the Prevention of Stroke in Subjects With Atrial Fibrillation

- A total of 18,201 patients with NVAF and at least 1 additional risk factor for stroke (mean $CHADS_2$, 2.1) were evaluated in a double-blind study comparing apixaban (5 mg twice daily [2.5 mg twice daily in high-risk patients]) with warfarin.
- The lower dose was used for those with 2 or more of the following factors associated with increased drug exposure: age greater than 80 years, body weight less than 60 kg, or serum creatinine level greater than 1.5 mg/dL. About 19% of these patients had a previous TIA, stroke, or systemic embolism.
- Apixaban was superior to warfarin in preventing stroke or systemic embolism (HR with apixaban, 0.79; 95% confidence interval [CI], 0.66–0.95; $P<.001$ for noninferiority; $P = .01$ for superiority).
- Apixaban also caused less bleeding and resulted in lower mortality (HR, 0.89; 95% CI, 0.80–0.99; $P = .047$) and reduced hemorrhagic stroke by 49% compared with warfarin ($P = <.001$).[16]

A Phase III Study of Apixaban in Patients With Atrial Fibrillation

- This trial compared apixaban and aspirin in 5599 patients with AF at increased risk for stroke unsuitable for VKA therapy.
- Apixaban reduced the risk of stroke or systemic embolism without significantly increasing the risk of major bleeding or intracranial hemorrhage.
- The trial was terminated early when apixaban was shown to be superior in reducing the risk of stroke or systemic embolism without increases in the risk of major bleeding or hemorrhagic stroke.[44]

Based on the results of the ARISTOTLE and AVERROES trials, apixaban has been approved for stroke prevention in patients with AF.

Global Study to Assess the Safety and Effectiveness of Edoxaban (DU-176b) vs Standard Practice of Dosing With Warfarin in Patients With Atrial Fibrillation

- This trial is the most recent and largest ever clinical trial on NOACs.
- This trial is of double-blind design, studying 21,105 patients who were randomized to receive edoxaban, 30 and 60 mg once daily, in comparison with warfarin for prevention of stroke in patients with AF.

- Both doses were halved if the patient had poor renal function (CrCl, 30–50 mL/min), weight 60 kg or less, or concomitant use of potent P-gp inhibitors (verapamil, quinidine, or dronedarone).
- Edoxaban 30 or 60 mg daily was noninferior to warfarin for the primary efficacy end point of stroke or systemic thromboembolism. However, in the intention-to-treat analysis, there was a trend favoring high-dose edoxaban versus warfarin ($P = .08$) and an unfavorable trend with low-dose edoxaban versus warfarin ($P = .10$).
- The rates of major bleeding including intracranial hemorrhage were significantly lower with both doses of edoxaban than with warfarin.
- Gastrointestinal bleeds were higher with high-dose edoxaban but lower with the low dose.[45]
- Based on these results, the drug is under consideration by the FDA for approval for the reduction in risk of stroke and systemic embolic events in patients with NVAF, as well as for the treatment of DVT or PE.

Study of the Safety, Tolerability and Pilot Efficacy of Oral Factor Xa Inhibitor Betrixaban Compared to Warfarin

- This trial is a phase 2, randomized, parallel-group, dose-finding multinational study of the safety, tolerability, and pilot efficacy of 3 blinded doses of betrixaban compared with open-label dose-adjusted warfarin in patients with NVAF with at least 1 risk factor for stroke.
- The primary end point was the time to major or clinically relevant nonmajor bleeding, and the secondary end point was time to any bleeding, death, stroke, myocardial infarction, or systemic embolism.
- The secondary objective was to study the pharmacokinetics of betrixaban.
- Betrixaban was well tolerated and had similar or lower rates of bleeding compared with well-controlled warfarin in patients with AF at risk for stroke.[46]

CLINICAL CONSIDERATIONS
Switching Between Anticoagulation Regimens

1. Switching to an NOAC: The aim is to minimize the risk of bleeding while maintaining the therapeutic effect during the transition between various drugs. While switching from warfarin to one of the newer anticoagulants, warfarin therapy may be stopped and NOAC therapy started when the INR is less than 2 in the case of dabigatran and apixaban and less than 3 in the case of rivaroxaban. For INR higher than these recommended values, the half-life of warfarin and the current INR should be taken into account to estimate when the INR value will likely drop to less than the threshold for the specific NOAC and a laboratory draw should be scheduled around that time. To switch from one NOAC to another, just substituting a new drug at the next dose should be considered. In switching from intravenous unfractionated heparin (UFH), the use of NOAC may be started 2 hours after heparin is discontinued, and in switching from low-molecular-weight heparin (LMWH), NOAC use may be initiated at the next due dose of LMWH. NOAC therapy can be started immediately after use of aspirin and clopidogrel is discontinued without waiting for the next due dose.

2. Switching from an NOAC: While switching to a VKA, it may take several days before an INR in the therapeutic range is obtained. Therefore, the NOAC should be administered concomitantly with the VKA until the INR is in a desired range. Owing to drug interactions between the 2 agents, it is advisable to test the INR just before the next intake of the NOAC during simultaneous administration and retest 24 hours after

the last dose of the NOAC. The INR should also be closely monitored for the first couple of months until stable values are reached. Use of heparin (UFH or LMWH) may be started when the next dose of NOAC is due.[47]

Dosing Errors

1. Missed doses: For NOACs with twice-daily and daily dosing regimens, a missed dose may be taken up till 6 and 12 hours, respectively, after the next scheduled dose, and subsequent dosing should be resumed as normal. If this is not possible, the dose should be skipped and the next dose should be taken at the scheduled time.
2. Double doses: For NOACs with a twice-daily regimen, the next planned dose should be skipped and twice-daily intake restarted in 24 hours. In daily dosing regimens, the normal regimen should be continued without skipping the next daily dose.
3. Uncertainty about dose: For twice-daily regimens, the planned dosing regimen could be continued without retaking the dose about which the patient was uncertain. For daily dosing regimens, another pill could be taken and then the planned dose regimen should be continued the next day.
4. Overdosing: Overdosing may occur intentionally or unintentionally or in the presence of concurrent events such as renal insufficiency. Depending on the clinical status and the amount of suspected overdose, the patient should be hospitalized. In case of overdose without bleeding, a wait-and-watch approach is reasonable given the short plasma half-life of NOACs. If the ingestion is recent, activated charcoal may be used to reduce absorption. Further management of bleeding is discussed- in the section on reversing anticoagulation effect.[47]

Reversal of Anticoagulation Effect

Reversal may be needed in the following situations:

1. Emergent surgical intervention: Attempts should be made to defer surgery for at least 12 hours, and ideally 24 hours, after the last dose. Evaluation of common coagulation tests as mentioned in **Table 3** may be undertaken if there is concern regarding waning in anticoagulation effect. The risk of bleeding is definitely increased and should be weighed against the urgency of intervention.
2. Management of bleeding complication: Specific antidotes and rapid (routine) quantitative measurements of anticoagulant effect are currently not available. Unlike in the case of VKAs, the plasma levels of NOACs may block newly administered coagulation factors. As the bleeding profile of NOACs, in particular that of intracranial and other life-threatening bleeding, is more favorable than that of warfarin, urgent restoration of coagulation may not be required in non–life-threatening bleeds. Restoration of coagulation does not necessarily equal good clinical outcome. In the case of dabigatran, activated charcoal may also be used for adsorbing drug from the stomach if ingestion has been recent, and hemodialysis may be used to remove dabigatran from the blood. **Fig. 3** outlines the management options in case of bleeding.[40,48–53]

Antidotes

1. A specific antidote for dabigatran has been developed and tested in animals but not yet in humans. The antidote has structural similarities with thrombin but an affinity for dabigatran that is about 350 times stronger than the affinity for thrombin. This antidote does not bind to known thrombin substrates and has no activity in coagulation tests or in platelet aggregation.[54]

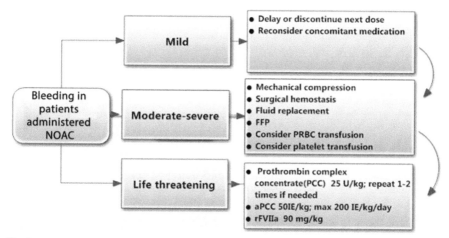

Fig. 3. Management of bleeding in patients administered NOACs. FFP, fresh frozen plasma; PRBC, packed red blood cells.

2. Betrixaban reversibility is being studied with andexanet alfa (PRT4445), an investigational recombinant fXa inhibitor antidote.[38]

Planned Surgery

1. Discontinuation of NOACs is not required for minor surgical procedures or those with a low bleeding risk. Procedures that carry a moderate to high risk of bleeding require a temporary interruption in the use of NOAC.[47,55,56]
2. Bridging was proposed in patients with AF with higher thromboembolic risk treated with VKAs but is not required in case of NOACs, as the predictable waning of the anticoagulation effect allows properly timed short-term cessation and reinitiation of NOAC therapy before and after surgery.
3. Although the aPTT and PT may provide a semiquantitative assessment of dabigatran and fXa inhibitors, respectively, it is not routinely recommended to aim at normalization of these clotting functions before surgery. Further information regarding specific categories is present in **Fig. 4**.

Atrial Fibrillation Ablation

1. AF ablations are considered high risk for bleeding because of the potential for multiple transseptal punctures and extensive case time. However, routine discontinuation of anticoagulation for 48 hours postprocedure is not advisable because of the high risk of thromboembolic complications immediately postprocedure.
2. There is controversy regarding the appropriate time to stop and start anticoagulation for AF ablations; Lakkireddy and colleagues[57] showed that NOACs given 24 hours before procedure and resumed within 3 hours following hemostasis were associated with a low complication rate, whereas Winkle and colleagues[58] advocated discontinuing NOACs for 36 hours before procedure and resuming at 22 hours postprocedure, with an interim bridge of 2 doses of enoxaparin (immediately and at 12 hours after ablation).
3. The VENTURE-AF study is following up 200 patients to prospectively evaluate the safety of rivaroxaban and VKAs around an AF ablation.[59]

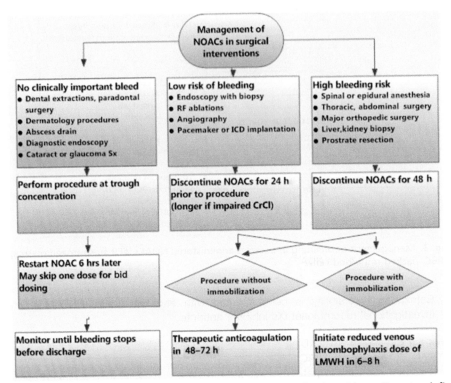

Fig. 4. Management of NOACs in surgical interventions. ICD, implantable cardioverter defibrillator; RF, radio frequency.

Cardioversion

1. In patients with AF of greater than 48 hours or unknown duration, oral anticoagulation should be therapeutic for at least 4 weeks before cardioversion, otherwise a transesophageal echocardiography (TEE) should be performed to rule out left-sided thrombi.[60]

2. After cardioversion, oral anticoagulation should be continued without interruption for another 4 weeks.

3. As there is no readily available coagulation assay for any of the NOACs, it is essential to establish and document compliance before cardioversion. A TEE should be performed if there are doubts about compliance.

4. In a subanalysis of the RE-LY trial, the frequencies of stroke and major bleeding within 30 days of cardioversion on both doses of dabigatran were low and comparable to those on warfarin, with or without TEE guidance.[61]

5. The X-veRT (Explore the Efficacy and Safety of Once-daily Oral Rivaroxaban for the Prevention of Cardiovascular Events in Subjects With Nonvalvular Atrial Fibrillation Scheduled for Cardioversion) trial showed that oral rivaroxaban not only was a safe and effective alternative to VKAs but also allowed earlier cardioversion compared with patients administered oral VKAs.[62]

POTENTIAL SOURCES OF ERROR IN NOVEL ORAL ANTICOAGULANT USE

The sources of error in **Fig. 5** may be seemingly obvious but have been the most common source of error and associated complications in NOACs use.

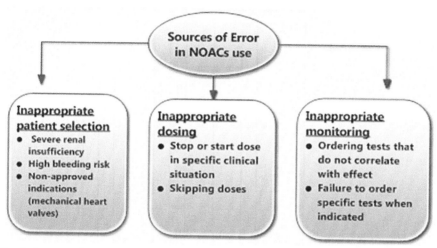

Fig. 5. Sources of error in NOAC use.

SPECIAL CONSIDERATIONS
Renal Failure

Chronic kidney disease (CKD) is associated with a relative increase in bleeding risk in patients administered NOACs. NOACs are, however, still a reasonable choice for anticoagulant therapy in patients with AF with mild or moderate CKD. Dabigatran, which is primarily cleared renally, may not be the NOAC of first choice in patients with known CKD, especially stage III or higher. A lower dose of dabigatran, at 75 mg twice daily, has been approved by the FDA for CrCl less than 30 mL/min. Dose reductions have been studied prospectively with apixaban (2.5 mg twice daily) and rivaroxaban (15 mg daily), and these may be more appropriate choices than dabigatran.[44,63] Renal function should be monitored at least every 6 months in patients with known renal dysfunction and yearly in patients with normal function at start of drug treatment. In the absence of clinical data or experience, NOAC therapy should be avoided in patients with AF who are on hemodialysis. VKAs may be a more suitable alternative, even though the benefit of VKAs in hemodialysis has not been proved.

Malignancy

Malignancy and AF occur in the elderly, and the use of NOACs in patients with malignancies is appropriate. Malignancies can predispose to stroke, and malignancies and their therapies are associated with a higher bleeding risk.[64] In all NOAC trials including Venous thromboembolism (VTE) trials, active malignancy was an exclusion criterion. When anticoagulant therapy needs to be initiated in a patient with malignancy, therapy with VKAs or heparins should be considered over NOACs, because of the clinical experience with these substances, the possibility of close monitoring, and reversal options. If the patient is on established anticoagulant therapy including NOACs when the malignancy is detected, the current anticoagulant should be continued whenever possible. Careful clinical monitoring for signs of bleeding and regular blood counts including platelets and liver and renal function must be performed.[47]

Table 5
Comparison of recent trials studying newer anticoagulants for secondary prevention of DVT/PE

Trial	RE-COVER	EINSTEIN-DVT	EINSTEIN-PE	AMPLIFY	HOKUSAI VTE	APEX
Drug	Dabigatran	Rivaroxaban	Rivaroxaban	Apixaban	Edoxaban	Betrixaban
Dose	150 mg bid	15 mg bid (3 wk) 20 mg Daily	15 mg bid (3 wk) 20 mg Daily	10 mg bid (1 wk) 5 mg bid (6 mo)	60 mg Daily	80 mg Daily
Control	Warfarin	Enoxaparin + warfarin	Enoxaparin + warfarin	Enoxaparin + warfarin	Enoxaparin or UFH + warfarin	Enoxaparin
Year	2008	2010	2011	2012	2013	2015 (estimate)
N	2564	3449	4832	5395	8250	6850 (estimate)
Study design	Double blind, double dummy	Randomized open label	Randomized open label	Randomized, double-blind study	Randomized, double-blind study	Double blind, double dummy
Age (mean) (y)	55	56	57.8	57	55.7	—
Women (%)	42	43	46	41	42.7	—
Prior VTE (%)	25.5	19	19	—	19	—
TTR (%)	59.9	57.7	62.7	61	63.5	—
Index event DVT	69	98.7	0	65	60	—
PE (%)	21	0	74.9	25.2	30	—
DVT&PE (%)	9.5	0.7	25.1	9.4	10	—

Duration of follow-up (mo)	7	3, 6, 12	3, 6, 12	7	12
Primary efficacy end point	VTE or related death	Recurrent VTE	Recurrent VTE	Recurrent VTE or death	VTE (DVT and/or PE) and VTE Death thro D35
Recurrent VTE HR	1.09	0.68	1.12	0.85	0.89
Major bleed HR	0.73	0.18	0.9	0.31	0.84
Clinically relevant nonmajor bleed HR	0.62	0.93	0.49	0.44	0.81
Death HR	1	0.67	1.13	0.79	1.05
Primary safety end point	Major bleeding, clinically relevant nonmajor bleed	Major bleeding, clinically relevant nonmajor bleed	Major bleeding, clinically relevant nonmajor bleed	Major bleeding, clinically relevant nonmajor bleed	Major bleeding, clinically relevant nonmajor bleed

Abbreviation: TTR, Time in therapeutic range.

AMPLIFY, Oral Apixaban for the Treatment of Acute Venous Thromboembolism; APEX, Acute Medically Ill VTE Prevention With Extended Duration Betrixaban Study; EINSTEIN-DVT, Oral Direct Factor Xa Inhibitor Rivaroxaban in Patients With Acute Symptomatic Deep Vein Thrombosis; EINSTEIN-PE, Oral Direct Factor Xa Inhibitor Rivaroxaban in Patients With Acute Symptomatic Pulmonary Embolism - The EINSTEIN PE Study; HOKUSAI VTE, Comparative Investigation of Low Molecular Weight (LMW) Heparin/Edoxaban Tosylate (DU176b) Versus (LMW) Heparin/Warfarin in the Treatment of Symptomatic Deep-Vein Blood Clots and/or Lung Blood Clots; RE-COVER, Efficacy and Safety of Dabigatran Compared to Warfarin for 6 Month Treatment of Acute Symptomatic Venous Thromboembolism.

NOVEL ORAL ANTICOAGULANTS IN DEEP VEIN THROMBOSIS/PULMONARY EMBOLISM

Although this article does not discuss the role of NOACs in PE and DVT in detail, highlights of the major trials studying the use of NOACs for DVT and PE are summarized in **Table 5**.[38,65–69]

SUMMARY

Based on efficacy, safety, and ease of use, NOACs will likely replace VKAs for many if not most patients with AF. Novel anticoagulants have a lower rate of intracranial hemorrhage compared with VKAs. The incidence of other life-threatening bleeds is similar if not lower. Dose adjustments need to be made based on renal function and advanced age. There is at present a need for an antidote for these new drugs.

REFERENCES

1. Wolf PA, Abbott RD, Kannel WB. Atrial fibrillation as an independent risk factor for stroke: the Framingham study. Stroke 1991;22:983–8.
2. Connolly SJ, Ezekowitz MD, Yusuf S, et al. Dabigatran versus warfarin in patients with atrial fibrillation. N Engl J Med 2009;361:1139–51.
3. Hirsh J. Oral anticoagulant drugs. N Engl J Med 1991;324:1865–75.
4. Camm AJ, Lip GY, De Caterina R, et al. 2012 Focused update of the ESC guidelines for the management of atrial fibrillation: an update of the 2010 ESC guidelines for the management of atrial fibrillation-developed with the special contribution of the European Heart Rhythm Association. Europace 2012;14(10):1385–413.
5. Skanes AC, Healey JS, Cairns JA, et al. Focused 2012 update of the Canadian Cardiovascular Society atrial fibrillation guidelines: recommendations for stroke prevention and rate/rhythm control. Can J Cardiol 2012;28(2):125–36.
6. Wann LS, Curtis AB, Ellenbogen KA, et al. 2011 ACCF/AHA/HRS focused update on the management of patients with atrial fibrillation (update on dabigatran): a report of the American College of Cardiology Foundation/American Heart Association Task Force on practice guidelines. J Am Coll Cardiol 2011;57(11):1330–7.
7. Dabigatran etexilate (Pradaxa)—a new oral anticoagulant. Med Lett Drugs Ther 2010;52:89–90.
8. Blech S, Ebner T, Ludwig-Schwellinger E, et al. The metabolism and disposition of the oral direct thrombin inhibitor, dabigatran, in humans. Drug Metab Dispos 2008;36:386–9.
9. Weinz O, Schwarz T, Kubitza D, et al. Metabolism and excretion of rivaroxaban, an oral, direct factor Xa inhibitor, in rats, dogs, and humans. Drug Metab Dispos 2009;37:1056–64.
10. Raghavan N, Frost CE, Yu Z, et al. Apixaban metabolism and pharmacokinetics after oral administration to humans. Drug Metab Dispos 2009;37:74–81.
11. Ogata K, Mendell-Harary J, Tachibana M. Clinical safety, tolerability, pharmacokinetics, and pharmacodynamics of the novel factor Xa inhibitor edoxaban in healthy volunteers. J Clin Pharmacol 2010;50(7):743–53.
12. Bathala MS, Masumoto H, Oguma T, et al. Pharmacokinetics, biotransformation, and mass balance of edoxaban, a selective, direct factor Xa inhibitor, in humans. Drug Metab Dispos 2012;40(12):2250–5.
13. Agnelli G, Buller HR, Cohen A, et al. Apixaban for extended treatment of venous thromboembolism. N Engl J Med 2013;368:699–708.

14. Bauersachs R, Berkowitz SD, Brenner B, et al. Oral rivaroxaban for symptomatic venous thromboembolism. N Engl J Med 2010;363:2499–510.
15. Cohen AT, Spiro TE, Buller HR, et al. Rivaroxaban for thromboprophylaxis in acutely ill medical patients. N Engl J Med 2013;368:513–23.
16. Granger CB, Alexander JH, McMurray JJ, et al. Apixaban versus warfarin in patients with atrial fibrillation. N Engl J Med 2011;15(36):981–92.
17. Patel MR, Mahaffey KW, Garg J, et al. Rivaroxaban versus warfarin in nonvalvular atrial fibrillation. N Engl J Med 2011;365(10):883–91.
18. Schulman S, Kearon C, Kakkar AK, et al. Dabigatran versus warfarin in the treatment of acute venous thromboembolism. N Engl J Med 2009;361:2342–52.
19. Schulman S, Kearon C, Kakkar AK, et al. Extended use of dabigatran, warfarin, or placebo in venous thromboembolism. N Engl J Med 2013;368:709–18.
20. Mueck W, Lensing AW, Agnelli G, et al. Rivaroxaban: population pharmacokinetic analyses in patients treated for acute deep vein thrombosis and exposure simulations in patients with atrial fibrillation treated for stroke prevention. Clin Pharmacokinet 2011;50:675–86.
21. Mendell J, Zahir H, Matsushima N, et al. Drug-drug interaction studies of cardiovascular drugs involving P-glycoprotein, an efflux transporter, on the pharmacokinetics of edoxaban, an oral factor Xa inhibitor. Am J Cardiovasc Drugs 2013; 13(5):331–42.
22. Wang L, Zhang D, Raghavan N, et al. In vitro assessment of metabolic drug-drug interaction potential of apixaban through cytochrome P450 phenotyping, inhibition, and induction studies. Drug Metab Dispos 2010;38:448–58.
23. Mendell J, Tachibana M, Shi M, et al. Effects of food on the pharmacokinetics of edoxaban, an oral direct factor Xa inhibitor, in healthy volunteers. J Clin Pharmacol 2011;51:687–94.
24. Kubitza D, Becka M, Zuehlsdorf M, et al. Effect of food, an antacid, and the H2 antagonist ranitidine on the absorption of BAY 59-7939 (rivaroxaban), an oral, direct factor Xa inhibitor, in healthy subjects. J Clin Pharmacol 2006;46: 549–58.
25. Stangier J, Stahle H, Rathgen K, et al. Pharmacokinetics and pharmacodynamics of the direct oral thrombin inhibitor dabigatran in healthy elderly subjects. Clin Pharmacokinet 2008;47:47–59.
26. Liesenfeld KH, Lehr T, Dansirikul C, et al. Population pharmacokinetic analysis of the oral thrombin inhibitor dabigatran etexilate in patients with non-valvular atrial fibrillation from the RE-LY trial. J Thromb Haemost 2011;9:2168–75.
27. Moore KT, Plotnikov AN, Thyssen A, et al. Effect of multiple doses of omeprazole on the pharmacokinetics, pharmacodynamics, and safety of a single dose of rivaroxaban. J Cardiovasc Pharmacol 2011;58:581–8.
28. Gnoth MJ, Buetehorn U, Muenster U, et al. In vitro and in vivo P-glycoprotein transport characteristics of rivaroxaban. J Pharmacol Exp Ther 2011;338: 372–80.
29. Mueck W, Kubitza D, Becka M. Co-administration of rivaroxaban with drugs that share its elimination pathways: pharmacokinetic effects in healthy subjects. Br J Clin Pharmacol 2013;76(3):455–66.
30. Lahaye SA, Gibbens SL, Ball DG, et al. A clinical decision aid for the selection of antithrombotic therapy for the prevention of stroke due to atrial fibrillation. Eur Heart J 2012;33:2163–71.
31. Stangier J, Rathgen K, Stahle H, et al. Coadministration of dabigatran etexilate and atorvastatin: assessment of potential impact on pharmacokinetics and pharmacodynamics. Am J Cardiovasc Drugs 2009;9:59–68.

32. Mendell J, Noveck R, Zahir H, et al. The effect of quinidine and verapamil, P glycoprotein/CYP3A4/5 inhibitors, on edoxaban pharmacokinetics and pharmacodynamics [abstract]. Basic Clin Pharmacol Toxicol 2010;107:2848.

33. Kubitza D, Mueck W, Becka M. No interaction between rivaroxaban - a novel, oral direct factor Xa inhibitor - and atorvastatin [abstract: P062]. Pathophysiol Haemost Thromb 2008;36:A40.

34. Stangier J, Stahle H, Rathgen K, et al. Pharmacokinetics and pharmacodynamics of dabigatran etexilate, an oral direct thrombin inhibitor, with coadministration of digoxin. J Clin Pharmacol 2012;52(2):243–50.

35. Kubitza D, Becka M, Zuehlsdorf M, et al. No interaction between the novel, oral direct factor Xa inhibitor BAY 59–7939 and digoxin [abstract: 11]. J Clin Pharmacol 2006;46:702.

36. Hartter S, Koenen-Bergmann M, Sharma A, et al. Decrease in the oral bioavailability of dabigatran etexilate after co-medication with rifampicin. Br J Clin Pharmacol 2012;74:490–500.

37. Hariharan S, Madabushi R. Clinical pharmacology basis of deriving dosing recommendations for dabigatran in patients with severe renal impairment. J Clin Pharmacol 2012;52(Suppl):119S–25S.

38. Cohen AT, Harrington R, Goldhaber SZ, et al. The design and rationale for the acute medically ill venous thromboembolism prevention with extended duration betrixaban (APEX) study. Am Heart J 2014;167(3):335–41.

39. van Ryn J, Baruch L, Clemens A. Interpretation of point-of-care INR results in patients treated with dabigatran. Am J Med 2012;125:417–20.

40. van Ryn J, Stangier J, Haertter S, et al. Dabigatran etexilate—a novel, reversible, oral direct thrombin inhibitor: interpretation of coagulation assays and reversal of anticoagulant activity. Thromb Haemost 2010;103:1116–27.

41. Huisman MV, Lip GY, Diener HC, et al. Dabigatran etexilate for stroke prevention in patients with atrial fibrillation: resolving uncertainties in routine practice. Thromb Haemost 2012;107:838–47.

42. Douxfils J, Mullier F, Robert S, et al. Impact of dabigatran on a large panel of routine or specific coagulation assays. Laboratory recommendations for monitoring of dabigatran etexilate. Thromb Haemost 2012;107:985–97.

43. Lindhoff-Last E, Samama MM, Ortel TL, et al. Assays for measuring rivaroxaban: their suitability and limitations. Ther Drug Monit 2010;32:673–9.

44. Connolly SJ, Eikelboom J, Joyner C, et al. Apixaban in patients with atrial fibrillation. N Engl J Med 2011;364(9):806–17.

45. Giugliano RP, Ruff CT, Braunwald E, et al, ENGAGE AF-TIMI 48 Investigators. Edoxaban versus warfarin in patients with atrial fibrillation. N Engl J Med 2013; 369(22):2093–104.

46. Connolly SJ, Eikelboom J, Dorian P, et al. Betrixaban compared with warfarin in patients with atrial fibrillation: results of a phase 2, randomized, dose-ranging study (Explore-Xa). Eur Heart J 2013;34(20):1498–505.

47. Heidbuchel H, Verhamme P, Alings M, et al. European Heart Rhythm Association. European Heart Rhythm Association Practical Guide on the use of new oral anticoagulants in patients with non-valvular atrial fibrillation. Europace 2013;15(5):625–51.

48. Stangier J, Rathgen K, Stahle H, et al. Influence of renal impairment on the pharmacokinetics and pharmacodynamics of oral dabigatran etexilate: an open-label, parallel-group, single-centre study. Clin Pharmacokinet 2010;49:259–68.

49. Levi M, Eerenberg E, Kamphuisen PW. Bleeding risk and reversal strategies for old and new anticoagulants and antiplatelet agents. J Thromb Haemost 2011; 9:1705–12.

50. Warkentin TE, Margetts P, Connolly SJ, et al. Recombinant factor VIIa (rFVIIa) and hemodialysis to manage massive dabigatran-associated postcardiac surgery bleeding. Blood 2012;119:2172–4.
51. Zhou W, Schwarting S, Illanes S, et al. Hemostatic therapy in experimental intracerebral hemorrhage associated with the direct thrombin inhibitor dabigatran. Stroke 2011;42:3594–9.
52. Eerenberg ES, Kamphuisen PW, Sijpkens MK, et al. Reversal of rivaroxaban and dabigatran by prothrombin complex concentrate: a randomized, placebo-controlled, crossover study in healthy subjects. Circulation 2011;124:1573–9.
53. van Ryn J, Ruehl D, Priepke H, et al. Reversibility of the anticoagulant effect of high doses of the direct thrombin inhibitor dabigatran, by recombinant factor VIIa or activated prothrombin complex concentrate. Haematologica 2008; 93(Suppl 1):148.
54. Schiele F, van Ryn J, Canada K, et al. A specific antidote for dabigatran: functional and structural characterization. Blood 2013;121(18):3554–62.
55. Healey JS, Eikelboom J, Douketis J, et al. Periprocedural bleeding and thromboembolic events with dabigatran compared to warfarin: results from the RE-LY randomized trial. Circulation 2012;126:343–8.
56. Sie P, Samama CM, Godier A, et al. Surgery and invasive procedures in patients on long-term treatment with direct oral anticoagulants: thrombin or factor-Xa inhibitors. Recommendations of the working group on perioperative haemostasis and the French study group on thrombosis and haemostasis. Arch Cardiovasc Dis 2011;104:669–76.
57. Lakkireddy D, Reddy YM, Di Biase L, et al. Feasibility and safety of dabigatran versus warfarin for periprocedural anticoagulation in patients undergoing radiofrequency ablation for atrial fibrillation: results from a multicenter prospective registry. J Am Coll Cardiol 2012;59(13):1168–74.
58. Winkle RA, Mead RH, Engel G, et al. The use of dabigatran immediately after atrial fibrillation ablation. J Cardiovasc Electrophysiol 2012;23:264–8.
59. Naccarelli GV, Cappato R, Hohnloser SH, et al, VENTURE-AF Investigators. Rationale and design of VENTURE-AF: a randomized, open-label, active-controlled multicenter study to evaluate the safety of rivaroxaban and vitamin K antagonists in subjects undergoing catheter ablation for atrial fibrillation. J Interv Card Electrophysiol 2014;41(2):107–16.
60. Fuster V, Rydén LE, Cannom DS, et al. 2011 ACCF/AHA/HRS focused updates incorporated into the ACC/AHA/ESC 2006 guidelines for the management of patients with atrial fibrillation: a report of the American College of Cardiology Foundation/American Heart Association Task Force on Practice Guidelines developed in partnership with the European Society of Cardiology and in collaboration with the European Heart Rhythm Association and the Heart Rhythm Society. J Am Coll Cardiol 2011;57(11):e101–98.
61. Nagarakanti R, Ezekowitz MD, Oldgren J, et al. Dabigatran versus warfarin in patients with atrial fibrillation: an analysis of patients undergoing cardioversion. Circulation 2011;123(2):131–6.
62. Cappato R, Ezekowitz MD, Klein AL, et al, X-VeRT Investigators. Rivaroxaban vs. vitamin K antagonists for cardioversion in atrial fibrillation. Eur Heart J 2014; 35(47):3346–55.
63. Fox KA, Piccini JP, Wojdyla D, et al. Prevention of stroke and systemic embolism with rivaroxaban compared with warfarin in patients with non-valvular atrial fibrillation and moderate renal impairment. Eur Heart J 2011;32: 2387–94.

64. Friberg L, Rosenqvist M, Lip GY. Evaluation of risk stratification schemes for is-chaemic stroke and bleeding in 182 678 patients with atrial fibrillation: the Swed-ish Atrial Fibrillation cohort study. Eur Heart J 2012;33:1500–10.
65. Schulman S, Kearon C, Kakkar AK, et al. Dabigatran versus warfarin in the treat-ment of acute venous thromboembolism. N Engl J Med 2009;361(24):2342–52.
66. EINSTEIN Investigators, Bauersachs R, Berkowitz SD, et al. Oral rivaroxaban for symptomatic venous thromboembolism. N Engl J Med 2010;363(26):2499–510.
67. EINSTEIN–PE Investigators, Büller HR, Prins MH, et al. Oral rivaroxaban for the treatment of symptomatic pulmonary embolism. N Engl J Med 2012;366(14): 1287–97.
68. Agnelli G, Buller HR, Cohen A, et al. Oral apixaban for the treatment of acute venous thromboembolism. N Engl J Med 2013;369(9):799–808.
69. Buller HR, Decousus H, Grosso MA, et al. Edoxaban versus warfarin for the treat-ment of symptomatic venous thromboembolism. N Engl J Med 2013;369(15): 1406–15.

Management of Atrial Fibrillation

Talal Moukabary, MD, Mario D. Gonzalez, MD*

KEYWORDS

- Atrial fibrillation • Ventricular rate • Sinus rhythm • Thromboembolism
- Catheter ablation • Antiarrhythmic drugs

KEY POINTS

- Management of atrial fibrillation includes the management of its risk factors and the underlying cardiac disease, prevention of thromboembolism, control of ventricular rate during atrial fibrillation, and restoration and maintenance of sinus rhythm.
- Prevention of thromboembolism should always be individualized to each patient.
- Control of ventricular rate during atrial fibrillation is essential for all patients.
- Restoration and maintenance of sinus rhythm are done through antiarrhythmic drug therapy, cardioversion, and catheter or surgical ablation.

INTRODUCTION

Atrial fibrillation (AF) is a very common clinical problem affecting more than 2.3 million US adults.[1] This high prevalence is expected to rise over time because of increasing risk factors (age, obesity, hypertension, and so forth).[1] About 35% of patients who are older than 80 years have AF.[2] This high prevalence is also associated with high cost because AF represents about 1% of overall health care spending.[3]

MANAGEMENT OF ATRIAL FIBRILLATION

The management of AF involves multiple facets: (1) management of underlying disease if present and the management of AF risk factors, (2) prevention of thromboembolism, (3) control of the ventricular rate during AF (rate control), and (4) restoration and maintenance of normal sinus rhythm (rhythm control).

MANAGEMENT OF THE UNDERLYING DISEASE AND RISK FACTORS

Management includes the treatment of modifiable predisposing or exacerbating factors including hypertension, obesity, heart failure, sleep apnea, and hyperthyroidism.

Clinical Electrophysiology, Penn State Heart and Vascular Institute, Milton S. Hershey Medical Center, Penn State University, 500 University Drive, Hershey, PA 17033, USA
* Corresponding author.
E-mail address: mgonzalez@hmc.psu.edu

Med Clin N Am 99 (2015) 781–794
http://dx.doi.org/10.1016/j.mcna.2015.02.007
0025-7125/15/$ – see front matter © 2015 Elsevier Inc. All rights reserved.

PREVENTION OF THROMBOEMBOLISM

Thromboembolism and stroke can have lethal or devastating consequences. This issue needs to be addressed in every patient with appropriate measures taken. The first step is assessment of the risk of thromboembolism. This risk is used to individualize the recommended therapy, and is based on clinical characteristics and not on whether AF is paroxysmal or persistent and regardless of whether or not AF is symptomatic.[2]

The following recommendations regarding anticoagulation for stroke and thromboembolism prevention are made in patients who have no contraindication for such therapy. Patients who have mechanical heart valves should be anticoagulated with warfarin.[2] Target international normalized ratio is 2 to 3 or 2.5 to 3.5 depending on valve type and location.[4]

Patients who have nonvalvular AF should be assessed using the CHA2DS2-VASc scoring system (Table 1).[5] Patients who have a CHA2DS2-VASc score of 2 or more should be considered for anticoagulation for stroke and thromboembolism prevention. This can be performed using warfarin therapy or with use of a direct thrombin or factor Xa inhibitor (dabigatran, rivaroxaban, or apixaban). Renal function is a major factor in choosing an agent for anticoagulation for stroke and thromboembolism prevention. Patients with end-stage renal disease are usually anticoagulated with warfarin.

Patients who have a CHA2DS2-VASc score of 1 may be treated with aspirin or warfarin or a direct thrombin or factor Xa inhibitor (dabigatran, rivaroxaban, or apixaban).[2] In patients who have a CHA2DS2-VASc score of zero it is reasonable not to use antithrombotic drug therapy.

Aspirin is usually prescribed as 325 mg by mouth daily, which is the dose that was used in the Stroke Prevention in Atrial Fibrillation trial.[6] This is the only study that showed benefit for aspirin alone in stroke prevention in patients with AF.[2]

Before prescribing aspirin, it is important to review the result of the Apixaban Versus Acetylsalicylic Acid to Prevent Strokes study,[7] which compared apixaban with aspirin in patients for whom vitamin K antagonist therapy was unsuitable. The study was prematurely terminated given the superiority of apixaban over aspirin in preventing stroke or systemic embolism, even though apixaban and aspirin had similar risk of major bleeding.[7]

When selecting the anticoagulant type and its dose it is critical to assess renal function and assess possible drug interactions. For an overview of the newer oral anticoagulants see Table 2.

Table 1
CHA2DS2-VASc scoring system for assessing thromboembolic risk in patients with nonvalvular atrial fibrillation

CHA2DS2-VASc Acronym	Score Points
Congestive heart failure	1
Hypertension	1
Age >75 y	2
Diabetes mellitus	1
Stroke/transient ischemic attack/thromboembolism	2
Vascular disease (prior myocardial infarction, peripheral vascular disease, aortic plaque)	1
Age 65–74 y	1
Sex category (ie, female sex)	1

Table 2 The newer oral anticoagulants		
Anticoagulant	**Mechanism of Action**	**Typical Dose[a]**
Dabigatran	Direct thrombin inhibitor	150 mg BID
Rivaroxaban	Direct factor Xa inhibitor	20 mg daily
Apixaban	Direct factor Xa inhibitor	5 or 2.5 mg BID[b]

[a] Typical dose for patients with normal renal function.
[b] Use apixaban 2.5 mg BID if any two patient characteristics present: creatinie ≥1.5 mg/dL, ≥80 y of age, body weight ≤60 kg.

Nonpharmacologic therapy for stroke and thromboembolism prevention involves left atrial appendage occlusion and excision. Percutaneous left atrial appendage occlusion can be performed using such devices as the WATCHMAN (Boston Scientific, Marlborough, MA). This device was shown to be noninferior compared with warfarin in patients who cannot receive warfarin.[8] Surgical excision of the left atrial appendage is usually performed for patients undergoing cardiac surgery for other indications.[2]

RATE CONTROL

Control of ventricular rate is an essential consideration in all patients with AF. Few patients do not need specific therapy for the control of ventricular rate during AF. This is usually related to an associated cardiac conduction system disease. This group of patients should be monitored because the progression of this conduction system disease may lead to symptomatic bradycardia.

It is not uncommon to see patients who have rapid ventricular rate during AF along with bradycardia during sinus rhythm caused by associated sinus node dysfunction. This is usually termed "tachycardia-bradycardia syndrome." However, the bradycardia that ensues after spontaneous or induced termination of AF may represent a transient functional sinus node dysfunction. If rhythm control of AF is not possible, some patients may require pacemaker therapy to avoid bradycardia and allow the use of rate control pharmacotherapy.

The target ventricular rate during AF was traditionally defined as having an average heart rate at rest less than or equal to 80 beats per minute and a maximum heart rate during a 6-minute walk test less than or equal to 110 beats per minute, or an average heart rate during 24-hour ambulatory electrocardiographic Holter monitoring less than or equal to 100 beats per minute (with no heart rate >110% maximum predicted age-adjusted exercise heart rate). This comes from the AFFIRM trial that showed that the management of AF with the rhythm-control strategy offers no survival advantage over the rate-control strategy.[9,10]

More recent data show that a more lenient strategy rate control (resting heart rate <110 beats per minute) can be as effective and easier to achieve.[11] This is a reasonable approach as long as the patient remains asymptomatic and the left ventricle function remains preserved.[2]

Pharmacotherapy to achieve rate control includes the use of blockers, nondihydropyridine calcium channel blockers, digoxin, and amiodarone. β-Blockers are frequently first-line therapy for rate control. They may not be tolerated well in patients with reactive airway disease. Nondihydropyridine calcium channel blockers are preferred in this group of patients.

Patients who have significant left ventricular systolic dysfunction may not well tolerate nondihydropyridine calcium channel blockers. In this group of patients cautious use of β-blockers is recommended. Another option for this group of patients is digoxin. Amiodarone is typically reserved as a second-line therapy given its side effect profile.

Patients with Wolff-Parkinson-White syndrome and pre-excitation should not be treated with atrioventricular nodal blocking agents because they may increase ventricular response and result in ventricular fibrillation.[2] This particular group of patients is best served by catheter ablation of the accessory pathway. **Table 3** provides a quick reference for selecting rate control agents.[2]

Atrioventricular junction ablation and pacing is an option used for patients who have advanced heart failure, rapid ventricular rate despite maximal drug therapy, and patients with advanced age or with poor prognosis and not candidates for catheter ablation of AF. It is typically a last resort option.

RHYTHM CONTROL
Cardioversion of Atrial Fibrillation

Cardioversion of AF can be done pharmacologically and electrically. Regardless of the method used for cardioversion, anticoagulation is a critical issue for prevention of stroke and thromboembolism. In patients who have been in AF for less than 48 hours and who are at low risk for thromboembolism, cardioversion can be performed with or without periprocedural anticoagulation.[2] In patients who have been in AF for less than 48 hours and who are at high risk for thromboembolism, anticoagulation should be initiated as soon as possible and continued after the cardioversion.[2]

Patients who have been in AF for more than 48 hours (or when the duration is unknown) should have been anticoagulated for a minimum of 3 weeks before the cardioversion. Anticoagulation should be continued after cardioversion for a minimum of 4 weeks in patients who are at low risk for thromboembolism and long term in those who are at high risk for thromboembolism.

In patients who cannot wait 3 weeks on anticoagulation before cardioversion, anticoagulation is initiated and once it is therapeutic, transesophageal echocardiogram is performed to rule out intracardiac thrombi. If no thrombi are found, cardioversion can be performed. Anticoagulation should be continued for a minimum of 4 weeks in patients who are at low risk for thromboembolism and long term in those who are at high risk for thromboembolism.

In patients who are hemodynamically unstable because of AF, cardioversion can be performed emergently along with starting anticoagulation. Anticoagulation should be

Table 3
Special considerations regarding drug choice for rate control

Clinical Condition	Drug of Choice	Caution
Reactive airway disease (asthma, chronic obstructive pulmonary disease)	CCB	β_1 selective β-blockers may be used with caution
Hypertension and HF with normal LV systolic function	β-blockers CCB	
LV systolic dysfunction with or without HF	β-blockers Digoxin	β-blockers should be used with caution as not to decompensate the HF
No other cardiovascular disease	β-blockers CCB	

Abbreviations: CCB, nondihydropyridine calcium channel blockers; HF, heart failure; LV, left ventricle.

continued for a minimum of 4 weeks in patients who are at low risk for thromboembolism and long term in those who are at high risk for thromboembolism. **Tables 4** and **5** summarize the recommendation for anticoagulation before and after cardioversion.

Pharmacologic cardioversion is performed using antiarrhythmic drug therapy. Ibutilide is a short-acting class III antiarrhythmic drug that is used specifically for cardioversion of AF. Care must be taken to ensure proper electrolyte balance, acceptable QT interval, and the absence of severe left ventricular dysfunction before using this drug. Given the potential for proarrhythmia, patients are electrocardiographically monitored during its use and for a minimum of 4 hours thereafter or until the QT returns to baseline. Defibrillation and advanced cardiac life support equipment and staff should be readily available.[2]

Oral antiarrhythmic drug therapies than can be used for cardioversion are flecainide, propafenone, dofetilide, and amiodarone. Flecainide and propafenone are contraindicated in patients with structural heart disease. Their use is usually preceded by administration of β-blockers or nondihydropyridine calcium channel blockers. This is to avoid conversion of AF to atrial flutter with 1:1 atrioventricular conduction, which can result in a very ventricular response (**Fig. 1**) or ventricular tachycardia/ventricular fibrillation. Dofetilide and amiodarone are discussed in more detail the next section.

Direct current cardioversion is a fast and effective way of cardioversion. However, it requires deep sedation or anesthesia and it offers no protection from the recurrence of AF. Strategies to prevent the recurrence of AF and maintain sinus rhythm include antiarrhythmic drug therapy and catheter ablation of AF.

Antiarrhythmic Drug Therapy

Antiarrhythmic drug therapy is usually first-line therapy for prevention of the recurrence of AF. Antiarrhythmic drugs are generally ion channel blockers. They are broadly classified as sodium channel blockers (or class I) and potassium channel blockers (or class III). Many drugs have a multichannel effect. They are only moderately effective and their use is limited because of their safety profile (**Table 6**).[9,12,13]

Potassium channel blockers delay repolarization resulting in prolonged action potential duration. This manifests as QT prolongation on the electrocardiogram and may cause torsades de pointes (**Fig. 2**).[14]

Sodium channel blockers can convert the AF to atrial flutter with 1:1 atrioventricular conduction resulting in very fast ventricular rate. This is a highly symptomatic arrhythmia that could result in syncope or death. Sodium channel blockers can result in atrioventricular block and bradycardia in patients with underlying conduction system disease. This bradycardia may result in torsades de pointes even in the absence

Table 4			
Anticoagulation for elective cardioversion			
Duration of Atrial Fibrillation	Thromboembolism Risk	Anticoagulation Before Cardioversion	Anticoagulation After Cardioversion
≤48 h	Low	Optional	Optional
≤48 h	High	Periprocedural	Long term
>48 h	Low	Minimum of 3 wk[a]	Minimum of 4 wk
>48 h	High	Minimum of 3 wk[a]	Long term

[a] Alternatively, anticoagulation can be initiated and once therapeutic a transesophageal echocardiogram can be performed and if no thrombi are present then cardioversion can be performed.

Table 5
Anticoagulation for emergent cardioversion

Duration of Atrial Fibrillation	Thromboembolism Risk	Anticoagulation Before Cardioversion	Anticoagulation After Cardioversion
<48 h	Low	Initiate immediately[a]	Optional
<48 h	High	Initiate immediately[a]	Long term
>48 h	Low	Initiate immediately[a]	Minimum of 4 wk
>48 h	High	Initiate immediately[a]	Long term

[a] Usually with heparin. Emergent cardioversion should not be delayed because of waiting for anticoagulation.

of potassium channel blockade. Sodium channel blockers can result in ventricular tachycardia or ventricular fibrillation in patients with structural heart disease.

With the exception of amiodarone and dofetilide no antiarrhythmic drug therapy can be used in patients with heart failure. Dronedarone can be used in patients who have coronary artery disease but not those who have advanced heart failure or recent heart failure exacerbation.[2]

Antiarrhythmic drug therapy is sometimes used in the early period after ablation. The early postablation period may have atrial arrhythmias that occur as a result of the ablation and they eventually resolve. This in itself does not imply failure of the ablation. Antiarrhythmic drug therapy can be used in this period to stabilize the rhythm. However, ablation is used in addition to antiarrhythmic drugs in patients who have failed antiarrhythmic drug therapy initially. The combination reduces the risk of recurrence of AF by half (91%–44%).[15]

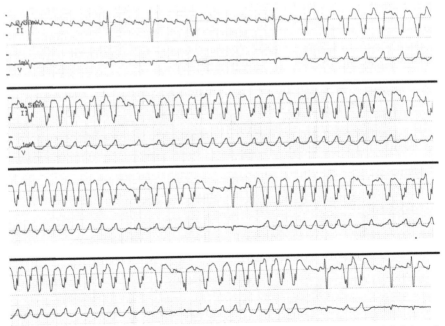

Fig. 1. Atrial flutter with intermittent rapid ventricular response associated with left bundle branch block aberrancy, simulating ventricular tachycardia.

Table 6
Commonly used drugs for antiarrhythmic drug therapy

Drug	Class	Exclude/Use with Caution	Major Pharmacokinetic Drug Interactions
Flecainide	Ic	Sinus or AV node dysfunction HF CAD Atrial flutter Infranodal conduction disease Brugada syndrome Renal or liver disease	Metabolized by CYP2D6 (inhibitors include quinidine, fluoxetine, tricyclics; also genetically absent in 7%–10% of population) and renal excretion (dual impairment can ↑↑plasma concentration)
Propafenone	Ic	Sinus or AV node dysfunction HF CAD Atrial flutter Infranodal conduction disease Brugada syndrome Liver disease Asthma Metabolized by CYP2D6 (inhibitors include quinidine, fluoxetine, tricyclics; also genetically absent in 7%–10% of population); poor metabolizers have ↑β blockade Inhibits P-glycoprotein: ↑digoxin concentration Inhibits CYP2C9: ↑warfarin	Inhibits most CYPs to cause drug interaction: ↑concentrations of warfarin (↑INR 0%–200%), statins, many other drugs Inhibits P-glycoprotein: ↑digoxin concentration
Amiodarone	III	Sinus or AV node dysfunction Infranodal conduction disease Lung disease Prolonged QT interval	Inhibits most CYPs to cause drug interaction: ↑concentrations of warfarin (↑INR 0%–200%), statins, many other drugs Inhibits P-glycoprotein: ↑digoxin concentration
Dofetilide	III	Prolonged QT interval Renal disease Hypokalemia Diuretic therapy Avoid other QT interval–prolonging drugs	Metabolized by CYP3A: verapamil, HCTZ, cimetidine, ketoconazole, trimethoprim, prochlorperazine, and megestrol are contraindicated; discontinue amiodarone at least 3 mo before initiation
Dronedarone	III	Bradycardia HF Long-standing persistent AF/flutter Liver disease Prolonged QT interval	Metabolized by CYP3A: caution with inhibitors (eg, verapamil, diltiazem, ketoconazole, macrolide antibiotics, protease inhibitors, grapefruit juice) and inducers (eg, rifampin, phenobarbital, phenytoin) Inhibits CYP3A, CYP2D6, P-glycoprotein: concentrations of some statins, sirolimus, tacrolimus, β-blockers, digoxin

(continued on next page)

Table 6 (continued)			
Drug	Class	Exclude/Use with Caution	Major Pharmacokinetic Drug Interactions
Sotalol	III	Prolonged QT interval Renal disease Hypokalemia Diuretic therapy Avoid other QT interval–prolonging drugs Sinus or AV nodal dysfunction HF Asthma	None (renal excretion)

Abbreviations: AV, atrioventricular; CAD, coronary artery disease; HCTZ, hydrochlorothiazide; HF, heart failure; INR, international normalized ratio.

Adapted from January CT, Wann LS, Alpert JS, et al. 2014 AHA/ACC/HRS guideline for the management of patients with atrial fibrillation: a report of the American College of Cardiology/American Heart Association Task Force on Practice Guidelines and the Heart Rhythm Society. Circulation 2014;130(23):e199–267; with permission.

Antiarrhythmic drugs, especially class Ic,can convert AF to atrial flutter.[16] In those patients, ablation of the resulting atrial flutter and continuing flecainide has 53% success at 5 years.

Catheter Ablation of Atrial Fibrillation

AF is frequently triggered by foci in the pulmonary veins (**Fig. 3**). Ablating those trigger foci inside the pulmonary veins may result in pulmonary vein stenosis. To decrease the chance of this complication, those triggers are typically treated by isolating the pulmonary veins outside the ostia. Other AF trigger sites are the superior vena cava, coronary sinus, and atrial walls. Catheter ablation of AF almost always includes pulmonary vein isolation. Based on clinical and electrophysiology findings, substrate modification is added.

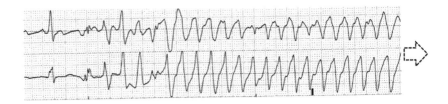

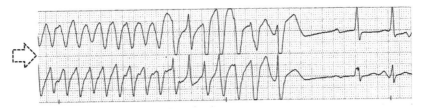

Fig. 2. Torsades de pointes during dofetilide administration.

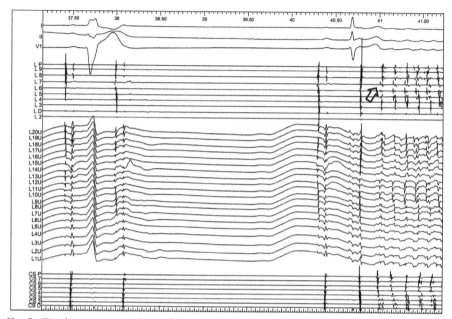

Fig. 3. Simultaneous recording of the electrocardiographic leads I, II, and V1 along with bipolar and unipolar electrograms recorded at the ostium of the left superior pulmonary vein as well as bipolar electrograms obtained from the coronary sinus (CS). Please note the strong vagal reaction followed by the onset of atrial fibrillation. The arrow depicts earliest electrical activity arising from the pulmonary vein.

Recurrence of Atrial Fibrillation After Ablation

Recurrence of AF after ablation can be related to reconnection of the pulmonary veins, persistent or new focal sources, and/or abnormal atrial substrate. Recurrence of AF is treated by ablation that focuses on reestablishing pulmonary vein isolation and ablation of focal sources.

In addition to reestablishing pulmonary vein isolation and ablation of focal sources, ablation of recurrent AF also includes treating the abnormal atrial substrate by creating lines of block between fixed anatomic obstacles (eg, the valves or other ablation lines) and ablation of sites of complex fractionated atrial electrograms during AF or sinus rhythm.

Typical Approach to Atrial Fibrillation Ablation

The initial ablation approach for treating paroxysmal AF is to ablate around the ostia of the pulmonary veins. Then, if there is recurrence of AF a more extensive ablation can be performed. This is to avoid the risks associated with extensive ablation, such as thromboembolism, proarrhythmia, and esophageal injury. The esophagus can be injured because of its close proximity to the posterior left atrial wall. Atrioesophageal fistula is a rare but nearly always fatal complication that happens because of such injury.

Persistent AF typically requires more extensive ablation compared with paroxysmal AF. Pulmonary vein isolation is still essential. However, in the case of persistent AF it is performed with a wide area circumferential ablation around pulmonary veins. This involves the atrial tissue more proximal to the ostia of the pulmonary veins.

Creating lines of block in the atrium can be used to eliminate macro reentrant atrial tachycardia. Those lines need to be complete otherwise they facilitate the induction of reentrant atrial tachycardias.

Even in highly experienced centered, serious complications can occur because of ablation, and ablation cannot eliminate AF in all patients.

Complications of Catheter Ablation

AF ablation requires extensive knowledge of the anatomy and electrophysiology of the atria and of transseptal cardiac catheterization techniques.[17] Catheter ablation–related mortality is 1 per 1000.[18] The main causes of death include cardiac tamponade, stroke, and atrioesophageal fistula.[18]

Cardiac tamponade frequency can potentially be reduced by careful transseptal access with use of intracardiac echocardiography. Another measure to decrease the frequency of cardiac tamponade is the gradual upward titration of radiofrequency (RF) energy during ablation. Perforation leading to tamponade happens in 1% of cases. It is usually treated with percutaneous pericardiocenthesis but it occasionally requires sternotomy or thoracotomy.[19]

The risk of stroke can potentially be reduced by proper anticoagulation and flushing of the transseptal sheath and by the use of irrigated tip ablation catheters.[20] Cerebrovascular accidents and transient ischemic attacks occur in about 1% of patients after AF ablation.

The risk of atrioesophageal fistula can potentially be reduced by the use of monitoring the intraluminal esophageal temperature and stopping ablation when the temperature rises. Another strategy is to reduce the RF energy when ablating the left atrial posterior wall.

Access site hematomas and pseudoaneurysms are a problem during catheter ablation. They are exacerbated by the need for anticoagulation for stroke prevention. Access site complications can potentially be reduced by the use of ultrasound-guided access.

Pulmonary vein stenosis is a well-known complication of AF. The risk is increased by ablating inside the pulmonary veins and is reduced by ablating outside the ostia. Use of three-dimensional mapping, cardiac computed tomography, cardiac MRI, and intracardiac echocardiography helps in reducing the frequency of pulmonary vein stenosis caused by inadvertent ablation inside the pulmonary veins. Pulmonary vein stenosis could be asymptomatic or could result in cough, dyspnea, chest pain, pulmonary infiltrate (localized pulmonary edema), and hemoptysis.

Micro or macro reentrant atrial tachycardias tend to develop in 3% to 40% of patients after AF ablation. The large variability in occurrence rate depends on ablation approach.[21–23] Macro reentrant atrial tachycardia is difficult to control with antiarrhythmic drug therapy and usual requires catheter ablation.

Phrenic nerve injury occurs in 0.1% to 0.48%. It is related to ablation in areas close to the phrenic nerves. Those areas are near the right superior pulmonary vein, left atrial appendage, and the superior vena cava.[24] This results in gastroparesis and its related symptoms. Phrenic nerve injury may be evident by fluoroscopy during ablation. It manifests as a decrease or cessation of movement of the corresponding part of the diaphragm. Before ablating areas that have a particularly high risk, such as the superior vena cava–right atrial junction, the operator can pace at high output from the location to test for phrenic nerve stimulation. Ablation should be avoided at areas where pacing stimulated the phrenic nerve. About 66% of patients with phrenic nerve injury after ablation do recover spontaneously.

Ablation Outcome

Recurrence of atrial fibrillation after ablation

Reconnection of the pulmonary veins is the most common cause of recurrence of AF. Inflammatory changes after ablation account for some arrhythmia. Recurrence of AF does not imply failure of the procedure. About 80% of isolated pulmonary veins reconnect at 4 months, although only 32% result in recurrence of AF.[25] Not all patients with pulmonary vein reconnection have recurrence of arrhythmia but most patients with recurrence of arrhythmia have at least partial reconnection in one or more of their pulmonary veins.

Silent AF is common after ablation. This has important significance because silent AF is asymptomatic but still poses a thromboembolic risk. Ablation improves quality of life even if it does not eliminate all forms of AF. After ablation, patients can feel the recurrence of AF only 75% of the time.[26] In the patients who have recurrence of symptoms, about 92% truly have recurrence of AF.[26]

Patients with paroxysmal AF who failed at least one antiarrhythmic drug have 16% chance of controlling AF with another antiarrhythmic drug compared with 66% by catheter ablation.[27] About 91.3% of patients with paroxysmal AF or persistent AF who were intolerant or failed two or more drugs have recurrence of AF. Only 44.1% have recurrence if treated with ablation plus antiarrhythmic drug therapy. Major complications occur in 4.4% of patients who have ablation.[15]

The Role of Pacing Without Atrioventricular Junction Ablation

Pacing helps prevent bradycardia. As such it allows use of antiarrhythmic drug therapy and atrioventricular nodal blocking agents. Atrial pacing prevents AF by preventing bradycardia and long pauses following premature atrial contractions. Patients with AF have paradoxic shortening of action potential duration after such long pauses. Bradycardia can result in torsades de pointes type ventricular arrhythmia especially in patients who are treated with antiarrhythmic drugs that prolong repolarization. Single-chamber atrial pacing or dual-chamber pacing is better than single-chamber right ventricular pacing.

Cryoballoon Ablation

Cryoballoon recently became available as a new way of performing AF ablation (**Fig. 4**). It provides circumferential ablation instead of the point-by-point ablation that is typically performed with RF ablation. It provides high acute success rate and a long-term success rate that is comparable with RF ablation. Cryoballoon

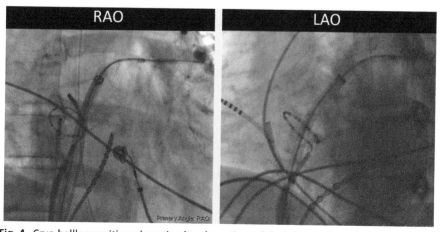

Fig. 4. Cryo-balllon positioned proximal to the ostium of the left superior pulmonary vein during cryo-ablation. RAO, right anterior oblique projection; LAO, left anterior oblique projection.

short-term success rate is reported to be 98%. Its long-term success is reported as 70% in patients with paroxysmal AF and 45% in patients with persistent AF.[28]

The concern about cryoballoon compared with the RF is the higher frequency of phrenic nerve injury reaching 6%. It occurs when ablating the right superior pulmonary vein. A strategy of pacing the phrenic nerve region while ablating that vein and stopping if there are signs of phrenic nerve paralysis has been used to decrease that complication. Other complications of cryoballoon are similar to RF and include pulmonary vein stenosis, stroke, tamponade, and groin hematoma. Initially it was thought that atrioesophageal fistulas would not occur with cryoballoon, but cases of that have been reported.

Surgical Ablation of Atrial Fibrillation

Surgical ablation of AF was initially the classic "cut and sew" Cox-Maze procedure. Success rate was reduced when that was replaced by ablation using RF, microwave, laser, and cryoablation.[29] Minimally invasive surgery can be done without the need for cardiopulmonary bypass. Patients who fail surgical ablation can undergo catheter ablation. Reasons for failure include incomplete isolation of the pulmonary veins, reconnection of the pulmonary veins, and triggers outside the lines of ablation created during surgery.

CURRENT DIFFICULTIES AND AREAS OF FUTURE DEVELOPMENT

At least part of the difficulty in managing AF is incomplete understanding of its pathophysiology. The main therapy options to help maintain normal sinus rhythm in patients who have AF are antiarrhythmic drug therapy and catheter ablation. Antiarrhythmic drug therapy has significant side effects that include causing new arrhythmias. Even if there are no side effects, antiarrhythmic drug therapy is associated with high AF recurrence rate.

The main target of catheter ablation of AF is pulmonary vein isolation. This ablation is mostly palliative. Only occasionally is it curative, usually in patients with localized triggers. It is not uncommon for AF to recur after catheter ablation. This is often caused by reconnection of the pulmonary veins or new triggers outside the veins. The treatment of recurrence is usually repeat catheter ablation.

Restoring and maintaining normal sinus rhythm with persistent AF is a more challenging task. Antiarrhythmic drug therapy is commonly ineffective, although drugs may be more effective after ablation. This is viewed as a success of catheter ablation because it allows a drug that failed previously to be successful in maintaining sinus rhythm.

REFERENCES

1. Go AS, Hylek EM, Phillips KA, et al. Prevalence of diagnosed atrial fibrillation in adults: national implications for rhythm management and stroke prevention: the AnTicoagulation and Risk Factors in Atrial Fibrillation (ATRIA) Study. JAMA 2001;285:2370–5.
2. January CT, Wann LS, Alpert JS, et al. 2014 AHA/ACC/HRS guideline for the management of patients with atrial fibrillation a report of the American College of Cardiology/American Heart Association Task Force on practice guidelines and the Heart Rhythm Society. Circulation 2014;130:e199–267 CIR.0000000000000041.
3. Lundqvist CB, Lip GY, Kirchhof P. What are the costs of atrial fibrillation? Europace 2011;13:ii9–12.
4. Nishimura RA, Carabello BA, Faxon DP, et al. ACC/AHA 2008 guideline update on valvular heart disease: focused update on infective endocarditis a report of the American College of Cardiology/American Heart Association Task Force on

practice guidelines: endorsed by the Society of Cardiovascular Anesthesiologists, Society for Cardiovascular Angiography and Interventions, and Society of Thoracic Surgeons. Circulation 2008;118:887–96.

5. Providencia R, Paiva L, Barra S. Risk stratification of patients with atrial fibrillation: biomarkers and other future perspectives. World J Cardiol 2012;4:195–200.

6. Stroke prevention in Atrial Fibrillation Study. Final results. Circulation 1991;84: 527–39.

7. Connolly SJ, Eikelboom J, Joyner C, et al. Apixaban in patients with atrial fibrillation. N Engl J Med 2011;364:806–17.

8. Reddy VY, Möbius-Winkler S, Miller MA, et al. Left atrial appendage closure with the watchman device in patients with a contraindication for oral anticoagulation: the ASAP Study (ASA Plavix Feasibility Study with Watchman left atrial appendage closure technology). J Am Coll Cardiol 2013;61:2551–6.

9. Wyse DG, Waldo AL, DiMarco JP, et al, Atrial Fibrillation Follow-up Investigation of Rhythm Management (AFFIRM) Investigators. A comparison of rate control and rhythm control in patients with atrial fibrillation. N Engl J Med 2002;347:1825–33.

10. Olshansky B, Rosenfeld LE, Warner AL, et al. The Atrial Fibrillation Follow-up Investigation of Rhythm Management (AFFIRM) study. Approaches to control rate in atrial fibrillation. J Am Coll Cardiol 2004;43:1201–8.

11. Van Gelder IC, Groenveld HF, Crijns HJ, et al. Lenient versus strict rate control in patients with atrial fibrillation. N Engl J Med 2010;362:1363–73.

12. Hohnloser SH, Kuck KH, Lilienthal J. Rhythm or rate control in atrial fibrillation–pharmacological intervention in atrial fibrillation (PIAF): a randomised trial. Lancet 2000;356:1789–94.

13. Van Gelder IC, Hagens VE, Bosker HA, et al. Rate control versus electrical cardioversion for Persistent Atrial Fibrillation Study Group: a comparison of rate control and rhythm control in patients with recurrent persistent atrial fibrillation. N Engl J Med 2002;347:1834–40.

14. Lazzara R. Antiarrhythmic drugs and torsade de pointes. Eur Heart J 1993; 14(Suppl H):88–92.

15. Stabile G, Bertaglia E, Senatore G, et al. Catheter ablation treatment in patients with drug-refractory atrial fibrillation: a prospective, multi-centre, randomized, controlled study (catheter ablation for the cure of Atrial Fibrillation Study). Eur Heart J 2006;27:216–21.

16. Ortiz J, Niwano S, Abe H, et al. Mapping the conversion of atrial flutter to atrial fibrillation and atrial fibrillation to atrial flutter. Insights into mechanisms. Circ Res 1994;74:882–94.

17. Cappato R, Calkins H, Chen SA, et al. Updated worldwide survey on the methods, efficacy, and safety of catheter ablation for human atrial fibrillation. Circ Arrhythm Electrophysiol 2010;3:32–8.

18. Cappato R, Calkins H, Chen SA, et al. Prevalence and causes of fatal outcome in catheter ablation of atrial fibrillation. J Am Coll Cardiol 2009;53:1798–803.

19. Cappato R, Calkins H, Chen SA, et al. Worldwide survey on the methods, efficacy, and safety of catheter ablation for human atrial fibrillation. Circulation 2005;111:1100–5.

20. Zhou L, Keane D, Reed G, et al. Thromboembolic complications of cardiac radiofrequency catheter ablation: a review of the reported incidence, pathogenesis and current research directions. J Cardiovasc Electrophysiol 1999;10:611–20.

21. Cummings JE, Schweikert R, Saliba W, et al. Left atrial flutter following pulmonary vein antrum isolation with radiofrequency energy: linear lesions or repeat isolation. J Cardiovasc Electrophysiol 2005;16:293–7.

22. Deisenhofer I, Estner H, Zrenner B, et al. Left atrial tachycardia after circumferential pulmonary vein ablation for atrial fibrillation: incidence, electrophysiological characteristics, and results of radiofrequency ablation. Europace 2006; 8:573–82.

23. Karch MR, Zrenner B, Deisenhofer I, et al. Freedom from atrial tachyarrhythmias after catheter ablation of atrial fibrillation: a randomized comparison between 2 current ablation strategies. Circulation 2005;111:2875–80.

24. Sacher F, Monahan KH, Thomas SP, et al. Phrenic nerve injury after atrial fibrillation catheter ablation: characterization and outcome in a multicenter study. J Am Coll Cardiol 2006;47:2498–503.

25. Cappato R, Negroni S, Pecora D, et al. Prospective assessment of late conduction recurrence across radiofrequency lesions producing electrical disconnection at the pulmonary vein ostium in patients with atrial fibrillation. Circulation 2003; 108:1599–604.

26. Neumann T, Erdogan A, Dill T, et al. Asymptomatic recurrences of atrial fibrillation after pulmonary vein isolation. Europace 2006;8:495–8.

27. Wilber DJ, Pappone C, Neuzil P, et al. Comparison of antiarrhythmic drug therapy and radiofrequency catheter ablation in patients with paroxysmal atrial fibrillation: a randomized controlled trial. JAMA 2010;303:333–40.

28. Andrade JG, Khairy P, Guerra PG, et al. Efficacy and safety of Cryoballoon ablation for atrial fibrillation: a systematic review of published studies. Heart Rhythm 2011;8:1444–51.

29. Stulak JM, Dearani JA, Sundt TM, et al. Superiority of cut-and-sew technique for the Cox maze procedure: comparison with radiofrequency ablation. J Thorac Cardiovasc Surg 2007;133:1022–7.

Indications for Pacemakers, Implantable Cardioverter-Defibrillator and Cardiac Resynchronization Devices

 CrossMark

Soraya M. Samii, MD, PhD

KEYWORDS

- Arrhythmia • Cardiac rhythm devices • Pacemaker
- Implantable cardioverter-defibrillator • Cardiac resynchronization therapy
- Systolic heart failure

KEY POINTS

- Patients with symptomatic inappropriate bradycardia from either sinus node dysfunction or atrioventricular (AV) block should be evaluated for a pacemaker.
- Patients who are asymptomatic with AV block and have heart rates less than 40 beats per minute or asystolic pauses greater than 3 seconds in sinus rhythm or greater than 5 seconds in atrial fibrillation WHILE AWAKE should be evaluated for a pacemaker.
- Patients who have symptomatic sustained ventricular tachycardia (VT) or ventricular fibrillation (VF) or have survived a cardiac arrest caused by VT/VF not from a reversible cause should be evaluated for implantable cardioverter-defibrillator (ICD).
- Patients who have chronic left ventricular (LV) systolic heart failure on guideline-directed medical therapy (GDMT) with an LV ejection fraction (EF) of 35% or less with New York Heart Association functional class II or III should be evaluated for ICD.
- Patients who have chronic LV systolic heart failure on GDMT with sinus rhythm and left bundle branch block and EF of 35% or less with QRS duration of 150 ms or greater should be evaluated for cardiac resynchronization therapy.

INTRODUCTION

Current guidelines for a particular field depend heavily on the history of the field. In the case of implantable cardiac rhythm devices, the way in which we categorize and establish appropriate use is structured on the history and evolution of these devices. In this article, the current implantable cardiac rhythm devices are described in their evolution and how the indications of these devices expanded over the decades.

Penn State Hershey Heart and Vascular Institute, Milton S. Hershey Medical Center, Penn State University, 500 University Drive, MC 047, Hershey, PA 17033, USA
E-mail address: ssamii@hmc.psu.edu

Med Clin N Am 99 (2015) 795–804
http://dx.doi.org/10.1016/j.mcna.2015.02.008
0025-7125/15/$ – see front matter © 2015 Elsevier Inc. All rights reserved.

medical.theclinics.com

The first implantable cardiac rhythm device was a pacemaker. This device was soon followed by the implantable cardioverter-defibrillator (ICD). Over time the utility in both was combined to provide both pacing and defibrillation in a single device. Both pacemakers and ICDs developed multi-chamber systems that could treat a combination of conduction disorders, heart failure, and tachyarrhythmias.

In this article, the indications and contraindications for device implantations are mainly extracted from the most current device guidelines from the American College of Cardiology Foundation/American Heart Association/Heart Rhythm Society, which were last revised in 2008 and then updated in 2012.

PACEMAKERS
History

The pacemaker was implanted in the first human in 1958. The concept of a permanent pacemaker was an extension of the very useful, yet primitive temporary pacemakers that proved to reduce mortality in the postoperative setting of congenital heart surgery in the early 1950s.[1] The initial experience with temporary pacemaker systems made it clear that some patients need indefinite pacing to survive. There were no randomized clinical trials during that era. However, clear benefits were inferred because of the known complications of untreated bradyarrhythmias, including syncope, ventricular arrhythmias, heart failure, and death. As the technology advanced with the development of transvenous leads, small battery design, and multi-chamber pacemakers with complex programming, the examination of utility and effectiveness of programming modes began to develop 1 to 2 decades after the initial invention. As it is now more than 60 years later, the data suggest the benefits in pacing are best in those with symptoms and those at high risk for conduction disease progression.[2] As pacemakers advanced to multi-chamber systems, their use in heart failure treatment is still evolving.

Persistent Bradycardia

There are 2 primary forms of sustained bradycardia: from sinus node dysfunction (SND) or atrioventricular (AV) block. There are no randomized clinical trials performed to show the benefit of pacemakers in this setting. A benefit has been observed with reduction in syncope and other symptoms associated with bradycardia and improved survival compared with those that do not receive a pacemaker.

Sinus Node Dysfunction

Patients who develop SND may present with inappropriate persistent bradycardia, episodic bradycardia, or chronotropic incompetence. The key feature of SND is that the bradycardia is inappropriate and not explained by normal physiology. It is important to make this distinction, as bradycardia during sleep or as a response to vagal tone, severe pain, or in the setting of physical training can be an appropriate response, with no symptoms and no indication for treatment.

Persistent inappropriate bradycardia can cause many symptoms, including dizziness, exertional symptoms, and syncope. The cause of SND is multifactorial but has been frequently described and simplified to be caused by fibrosis or aging of the sinus node. Evaluations of the atrium in those with SND clearly show structural remodeling that supports this simplified theory.[3] At the same time, there are normal changes to the sinus node with age that also contribute to the cause of SND.[4] These changes have been described in greater detail to include changes in ion channel expression clearly giving evidence that the description of fibrosis is a greatly simplified theory.[5] The presentation of SND is most dramatically described with syncope. Other presentations may be more subjective with dizziness, weakness, and fatigue as the heart rate does not respond appropriately to the activities of daily living resulting in depressed cardiac output. When SND is left untreated with the clinical presentation of syncope, there is frequently recurrent syncope. The diagnosis of SND can be variable if there is not symptomatic persistent bradycardia. Further testing is usually warranted, including long-term rhythm monitoring with Holter, event recorder, exercise testing, and implantable loop recorder to correlate the bradycardia with symptoms.

Indications and Contraindications for Pacing with Sinus Node Dysfunction

A permanent pacemaker for SND is indicated with documented symptomatic bradycardia and chronotropic incompetence that is not reversible with medicine changes. Pacing is also indicated with these findings when drug therapy that may be contributing to the bradycardia is required for treatment of medical conditions.[2] Pacemaker placement is not indicated for SND when there are no symptoms. Pacing is also not indicated when the symptoms have been proven not to be caused by bradycardia.[2]

In patients who have SND requiring a pacemaker, the risk of those patients developing AV block and requiring a ventricular lead over time has been measured at 1.7% per year in a clinical trial.[6] This finding has been consistent in other observational studies.[7] Dual-chamber pacemakers are, therefore, most commonly placed for this indication. Occasionally single-chamber atrial pacing systems are placed in individuals who are not as likely to progress with AV block.

Atrioventricular Block

AV block is typically described as block in the AV node, bundle of His, or below the bundle of His. It is also clinically interpreted as type I, type II or type III AV block that often correlates with the specific site of block. The AV block may be intermittent or persistent. There may also be transitions from one type of block to another, especially if there is coincident conduction disease below the AV node. In type III AV block, there is a complete block of the electrical impulse at or below the bundle of His with no conduction from the atrium to the ventricle. The result is an escape rhythm most frequently originating from the ventricle that is not dependable long-term. Patients with this condition may be symptomatic from the slow rhythm or from induction of ventricular arrhythmias. Early observational studies have demonstrated improvement of symptoms and survival with pacemakers.[7]

In the case of type I or type II heart block, the decision of pacemaker placement depends on the degree of symptoms and concern for progression to more advanced heart block. Certainly if there are symptoms associated with bradycardia or loss of appropriate AV synchrony, dual-chamber pacing will improve symptoms. If there are no symptoms further diagnostic evaluation is recommended to determine if the site of the block is above or below the AV node and if there is risk of developing further conduction disease. If the electrocardiogram demonstrates conduction disease in the bundles with bifascicular block or left bundle branch block (LBBB), there is clear concern for progression of AV block to more advanced heart block. Studies may include a diagnostic electrophysiologic study, stress testing, or long-term monitoring.

In the setting of AV block, there is the need to evaluate for potential reversible causes. One such example would be for Lyme infection causing heart block in a young person. Treatment in this example would be with antibiotics and supportive care without the need for long-term permanent pacing. Another reversible cause of AV block would be drug toxicity. In addition to looking for reversible causes, there is often the need to evaluate patients with AV block for associated comorbidities. This evaluation may involve performing other cardiac testing to exclude other associated cardiac comorbidities, such as heart failure, ischemic heart disease, valvular heart disease, or sustained ventricular arrhythmias. There may also need to be an evaluation for more systemic illnesses, such as sarcoidosis or amyloidosis.

Indications and Contraindications for Pacing with Atrioventricular Block

Implantation of a permanent pacemaker should always be considered in those with any type of AV block when it is proven that symptoms are related to the conduction abnormality. Symptoms could be caused by the bradycardia or the ventricular arrhythmias caused by the bradycardia. A pacemaker should also be considered in these situations when patients are symptomatic and yet require drug therapy that results in the symptomatic bradycardia. Pacemakers should be considered even without symptoms when there is concern that the conduction abnormality can worsen. Such signs of risk of progression include evidence of alternating bundle branch block or asystolic pauses in awake individuals of 3 seconds or more during sinus rhythm or 5 seconds or more in atrial fibrillation.[2] Pacemakers should also be considered in those with any escape rhythm less than 40 beats per minute while awake.[2]

Pacemakers are not indicated in asymptomatic individuals who demonstrate AV block above the AV node without coincident conduction disease, such as LBBB or bifascicular block. Pacemakers are not indicated in situations where the AV block is expected to be transient and not likely to recur as in the cases of drug toxicity or Lyme infection.[2]

Most pacemakers placed for AV block are dual chamber pacemakers to maintain AV synchrony. The exception to this would be in those patients with permanent atrial fibrillation where only ventricular pacing is required. Dual-chamber pacemaker systems have shown to have fewer incidences of atrial fibrillation and pacemaker syndrome compared with ventricular pacing systems.[8] There has been no benefit in regard to mortality or heart failure progression between dual-chamber pacing and ventricular pacing systems.[9]

The result of pacemaker placement in the setting of AV block will be right ventricular (RV) pacing. In early pacing studies, RV pacing did not alter long-term heart failure progression.[9] It is now evident that RV pacing may also accelerate the heart failure process in those with depressed left ventricular (LV) systolic function.[10,11] The potential detrimental effects of chronic RV pacing may lead to worsening LV systolic heart failure. The current updated 2012 guidelines for device-based therapy recommend consideration of cardiac resynchronization therapy (CRT) in patients with LV ejection fraction (LVEF) of 35% or less when anticipated ventricular pacing is expected to be greater than 40%.[12] This recommendation may change with future revisions with new data suggesting that CRT may benefit those with only mild LV systolic impairment. In the Biventricular Pacing for AV Block and Systolic Dysfunction (BLOCK HF) trial, patients who required ventricular pacing because of heart block or very prolonged first-degree heart block were randomized to either a dual-chamber pacemaker or CRT pacing if the LVEF was 50% or less. CRT in this trial showed a significant reduction in heart failure hospitalizations with a hazard ratio −0.70 (confidence interval 0.52–0.93).[13]

Atrial Fibrillation

Pacemakers are indicated for atrial fibrillation when there is a slow ventricular response associated with symptoms. Pacemakers are also indicated in atrial fibrillation when there are pauses of greater than 5 s while patients are awake or symptomatic termination pauses.[2] Pacemakers should be considered even when medicines are causing the slow heart rhythm if the medicines are required to control either the rhythm or rate of the atrial fibrillation.

Single-chamber ventricular pacing systems are placed in those with permanent atrial fibrillation. In individuals with paroxysmal atrial fibrillation, a dual-chamber pacemaker is often implanted to promote AV synchrony during sinus rhythm, if required. In patients with difficult-to-control atrial fibrillation with rapid ventricular response, a pacemaker may be placed in preparation for an AV junction ablation.[2]

When patients have coincident LV systolic dysfunction with an LVEF of 35% or less with anticipated pacing of more than 40% or if there is coincident LBBB, a CRT pacing system may be considered to reduce the heart failure progression and heart failure hospitalization.[12]

Neurocardiogenic Syndromes

Neurocardiogenic syndromes account for most cases of syncope in the general population.[14] These syndromes have a spectrum that includes hypersensitive carotid sinus syndrome (HCS), neurocardiogenic syncope (NS), orthostatic intolerance, and postural orthostatic tachycardia syndrome. Despite the high frequency of syncope and near syncope in these conditions, pacemakers are only rarely indicated.

In the case of HCS, it is a diagnosis given to those that demonstrate an exaggerated reflex response to carotid sinus stimulation. Both normal and exaggerated carotid sinus stimulation can involve a cardioinhibitory reflex and a vasodepressor reflex or a combination of both. Both components are caused by increases in parasympathetic tone or decreases in sympathetic tone from carotid sinus stimulation. With the cardioinhibitory response, there can be transient slowing of the sinus rate and slowing of AV node conduction causing slowing of the heart rate, increasing PR interval, and sometimes transient AV block. The vasodepressor component is a result of a reduction in vascular tone that causes transient hypotension. Either of these components can result in near syncope or syncope. When both components occur, there is a greater chance of symptoms. A permanent pacemaker may be considered when recurrent spontaneous carotid hypersensitivity results in recurrent syncope and there is a profound cardioinhibitory response with ventricular asystole greater than 3s with carotid sinus pressure.[15]

In the case of NS, there is a reflex that can be triggered by a variety of scenarios that can cause a vasodepressor or cardioinhibitory response. Such scenarios include prolonged standing, pain, anxiety, and stress. Frequently these events result in a combination of both a component of transient hypotension and bradycardia. Permanent pacing in this condition has not been shown to significantly reduce recurrent syncope.[16] Pacemakers should not be considered a first-line treatment of this condition.[2]

Other Conditions that Require Pacing

There are several familial and acquired disorders that may require pacemaker placement because of the risk of conduction disease progression or to minimize the risk of tachyarrhythmia. Examples of inherited conditions include neuromuscular disorders that have been associated with progressive conduction disease. Some forms of long QT syndrome may also require pacing in individuals that continue to have symptoms despite treatment with beta-blockers. Acquired conditions include cardiac sarcoidosis that can result in conduction disease progression and frequently require evaluation for a pacemaker.[2]

IMPLANTABLE CARDIOVERTER-DEFIBRILLATOR
History

Similar to the invention of the permanent pacemaker, the concept of an implantable standby defibrillator emerged from the observation that individuals with coronary artery disease with recurrent symptomatic ventricular tachycardia (VT) were at high risk for dying suddenly.[17] Ten years later, the first ICD was implanted successfully in 3 patients who had demonstrated malignant ventricular arrhythmias.[18,19] This success led to the first trial to test the benefit of the ICD. In 1985, the Food and Drug Administration approved the first of what would be many indications for ICD implantation.[20] Initially, the only approved indications for ICD placement were in individuals who had survived a cardiac arrest or demonstrated significant symptoms from sustained ventricular fibrillation (VF) or VT.

The current indications for ICD implantation are reviewed later. There are also major contraindications to ICD placement even if the individual has an otherwise qualifying indication. ICD placement is contraindicated in patients who do not have anticipated survival beyond 1 year or have New York Heart Association (NYHA) functional class IV that do not qualify for CRT or transplant. ICD therapy may be contraindicated because of "significant psychiatric illnesses that may be aggravated by device implantation" or follow-up.[2] An ICD implant would not be recommended in any patient with ongoing systemic infection. ICD placement is not effective in individuals with uncontrolled ventricular arrhythmias.[2]

Secondary Prevention of Sudden Death

Following the feasibility of ICD implantation with successful standby defibrillator function in the 1980s, there was a need to prove the benefit of the implantation against the risk of the procedure. The benefit of the ICD technology in a small high-risk population was the launching pad for several larger randomized controlled clinical trials in the next decade to further prove the effectiveness of the ICD in the secondary prevention of sudden cardiac death (SCD). A meta-analysis of the 3 largest trials evaluating the utility of ICD therapy in secondary prevention demonstrated a 28% reduction in all-cause mortality with the ICD compared with those treated with antiarrhythmic medications.[21]

Indications and Contraindications for Implantable Cardioverter-Defibrillator Placement for Secondary Prevention of Sudden Cardiac Death

Individuals who survive a cardiac arrest caused by sustained VT or VF that is not from a reversible cause should be considered for ICD implantation. Exclusions would include an anticipated life expectancy of less than 1 year, uncontrolled ventricular arrhythmias, or a defined completely reversible cause of the VT or VF episode. Patients with spontaneous sustained VT and structural heart disease should be considered for ICD. Patients with syncope and sustained ventricular arrhythmias during electrophysiologic study should be considered for ICD placement.[2]

Primary Prevention of Sudden Death

The large benefit in this still relatively small population of individuals who had demonstrated and survived sustained VT or VF raised 2 questions: (1) whether it was possible to identify a population of patients before their first episode of a sustained ventricular arrhythmia and (2) whether these individuals would also benefit from ICD therapy. From this concept, more randomized clinical trials were designed to evaluate for a benefit of ICD therapy in patients at high risk for sudden death. The initial trials evaluating the benefit for primary prevention of sudden death were focused on the population with a history of myocardial infarction (MI), coronary artery disease, and LVEF. In the largest of these trials, the Multicenter Automatic Defibrillator Implantation Trial II (MADIT II), there was a 31% reduction in all-cause mortality compared with the control group.[22] The difference was so significant early in the trial that the trial was stopped at 20 months of follow-up because of the improved survival rates in the ICD arm.[23]

Once the results clearly defined a benefit from ICD therapy in individuals with a history of MI and reduced LVEF, the focus moved to evaluate individuals with heart failure resulting from chronic LV systolic dysfunction. The largest randomized clinical trial for primary prevention was launched: Sudden Cardiac Death in Heart Failure Trial (SCD-HefT). This trial enrolled individuals with chronic systolic heart failure who were on optimal medical therapy for at least 3 months before enrollment and continued to have an LVEF of 35% or less. In this trial, there was a 23% reduction in mortality in those randomized to ICD with an LVEF of 35% or less with NYHA functional status II or III.[24] In those with less symptomatic heart failure symptoms with NYHA class II functional class, the reduction in mortality with an ICD was calculated as high as 46%.[24]

Indications for Primary Prevention of Sudden Cardiac Death

ICD therapy has been shown to benefit patients with an LVEF of 35% or less with NYHA functional class II or III on optimal medical therapy more than 40 days following MI. Individuals with a history of MI, NYHA functional class I, and an LVEF less than 30% should also be considered for ICD. ICD therapy should be considered in patients with nonischemic cardiomyopathy with an EF of 35% or less with NYHA functional class II or III on optimal medical therapy for more than 3 months.[2]

There are also rare and/or inherited conditions that may be identified as high risk for sudden death. Some of these situations should be considered for ICD for the primary prevention of sudden death. Examples include patients with hypertrophic cardiomyopathy with multiple high-risk features.[2] Some forms of long QT, Brugada, and arrhythmogenic RV dysplasia are some examples of high-risk inherited disorders.[2] It is common with these syndromes that a family member has died suddenly or received and ICD as a secondary prevention indication.

There are clear contraindications to ICD placement even when there are criteria supporting ICD placement. Situations whereby ICD therapy would not be indicated include patients who do not have a the expected survival of more than 1 year, patients with a poor functional class defined as NYHA class IV who are not eligible for transplant, and patients with a severe psychiatric illness that may be made worse by implantation or interfere with the required follow-up.[2]

CARDIAC RESYNCHRONIZATION THERAPY
History

More than 3 decades after the first implanted permanent pacemaker, it is clear that pacing does not improve heart failure outcomes.[9] There has been growing evidence that a widened QRS complex correlated with increased mortality.[25] The widened QRS created by RV pacing may explain the lack of improvement in heart failure from dual-chamber pacing for AV block. A theory evolved from these observations that contractility may improve with a narrow QRS.[26] In the mid 1990s, biventricular pacing improving transient hemodynamics was reported in patients with heart failure and wide QRS duration.[27] From here, multiple randomized controlled trials were launched to further evaluate the benefit of multisite pacing that would later be termed CRT in the chronic systolic heart failure population with prolonged QRS duration.

Cardiac Resynchronization Therapy for Symptomatic Systolic Heart Failure

In 2001, the first multicenter randomized controlled clinical trial of CRT was published with results demonstrating feasibility, improved exercise tolerance, and quality of life in patients with advanced heart failure and QRS complexes greater than 150 ms.[28] This trial was followed by several larger randomized prospective controlled trials in patients with symptomatic heart failure that further supported CRT in heart failure management.[29–31] Some trials also included the evaluation of ICD in the same population. As discussed in the section regarding the primary prevention of SCD, this population with chronic systolic heart failure would benefit from ICD therapy. In the Comparison of Medical Therapy, Pacing, and Defibrillation in Heart Failure (COMPANION) trial, there was a 24% relative risk reduction in all-cause mortality in patients with advanced heart failure with CRT pacing compared with optimal medical therapy.[31] The reduction in morality was even greater with a CRT and ICD (CRTD) combination device with a 36% relative risk reduction in all-cause mortality at 1 year.[31] In another large European trial of CRT, patients with advanced systolic chronic heart failure and wide QRS receiving a CRT pacemaker had a 36% relative risk reduction in mortality compared with those treated medically.[30] In large retrospective evaluations of patients with CRT therapy, there were better outcomes in those with LBBB morphology at baseline than those with non-LBBB prolonged QRS intervals.[32,33]

Cardiac Resynchronization Therapy for Less Symptomatic Systolic Heart Failure

With these exciting results in patients with symptomatic heart failure, there was a move to offer CRT to patients with less symptomatic systolic heart failure with NYHA class II functional status, low EF, and wide QRS duration. The Multicenter Automatic Defibrillator Implantation Trial with Cardiac Resynchronization Therapy (MADIT-CRT) trial evaluated less symptomatic NYHA class I and II functional class with an LVEF of 30% or less and QRS durations of 130 ms or greater. This trial was unique in that all patients in the trial received an ICD. In those who received CRTD, there was a 34% reduction in the primary end point of heart failure hospitalization or death.[34] The benefit was mainly driven by a 41% reduction in heart failure hospitalization as all patients received an ICD.[34] The benefit of reduced heart failure events with CRT was higher in those with QRS durations of 150 ms or greater.

Indications for Cardiac Resynchronization Therapy

CRT with or without ICD should be considered in patients who have chronic LV systolic heart failure with NYHA functional class II, III, or ambulatory IV, sinus rhythm and LBBB with QRS duration of 150 ms or greater and LVEF of 35% or less on guideline-directed medical therapy (GDMT). CRT may be considered in patients with more symptomatic NYHA functional class III and ambulatory IV heart failure with an LVEF of 35% or less (on GDMT) when the LBBB QRS duration is 120 to 149 ms or a non-LBBB QRS duration of 150 ms or greater.[12]

With the evidence of reduction in heart failure events with CRT, indications for CRT have also been expanded to be considered in most RV pacing indications in the setting of systolic heart failure with an EF of 35% or less (on GDMT) when RV pacing is expected to be more than 40%. Potential candidates would include patients with atrial fibrillation who require ventricular pacing (including those who have had AV nodal ablation).[12]

As with all implantable cardiac rhythm devices, there are clear contraindications to CRT even if the criteria for placement are present. The most recent update to the guidelines clarified the class III recommendation whereby the procedure is not recommended in "patients in whom cardiac and noncardiac comorbidity and/or frailty limit survival with good functional capacity to less than 1 year."[12]

SUMMARY

Implantable cardiac rhythm devices have become an important part of our management of patients with heart rhythm disorders. The tools and indications have evolved since that first implantable device in a man with complete heart block more than 50 years ago. There will continue to be evolution of indications and guidelines with these important tools.

REFERENCES

1. Weirich WL, Gott VL, Lillehei CW. The treatment of compete heart block by the combined use of a myocardial electrode and an artificial pacemaker. Surg Forum 1958;8:360–3.
2. Epstein AE, Dimarco JP, Ellenbogen KA, et al. ACC/AHA/HRS 2008 guidelines for device-based therapy of cardiac rhythm abnormalities: a report of the American College of Cardiology/American Heart Association task force on practice guidelines. J Am Coll Cardiol 2008;51:e1–62.
3. Sanders P, Morton JB, Kistler PM, et al. Electrophysiological and electroanatomic characterization of the atria in sinus node disease: evidence of diffuse atrial remodeling. Circulation 2004;109:1514–22.
4. Kistler PM, Sanders P, Fynn SP, et al. Electrophysiologic and electroanatomic changes in the human atrium associated with age. J Am Coll Cardiol 2004;44:109–16.
5. Jones SA, Boyett MR, Lancaster MK. Declining into failure: the age-dependent loss of the L-type calcium channel within the sinoatrial node. Circulation 2007;115:1183–90.
6. Nielsen JC, Thomsen PE, Hojberg S, et al. A comparison of single-lead pacing with dual-chamber pacing in sick sinus syndrome. Eur Heart J 2011;32:686–96.
7. Brignole M, Auricchio A, Baron-Esquivias G, et al. 2013 ESC guidelines of cardiac pacing and cardiac resynchronization therapy. Europace 2013;15:1070–118.
8. Healey JS, Toff WD, Lamas GA, et al. Cardiovascular outcomes with atrial-based pacing compared with ventricular pacing. Circulation 2006;114:11–7.
9. Toff WD, Camm AJ, Skehan JD, et al. Single-chamber versus dual-chamber pacing for high-grade atrioventricular block. N Engl J Med 2005;353:145–55.
10. Wilkoff BL, Kudenchuk PJ, Buxton AE, et al. The DAVID (Dual Chamber and VVI Implantable defibrillator) II trial. J Am Coll Cardiol 2009;53:872–80.
11. Barsheshet A, Moss AJ, McNitt S, et al. Long-term implications of cumulative right ventricular pacing among patients with an implantable cardioverter-defibrillator. Heart Rhythm 2011;8:212–8.
12. Tracy CM, Epstein AE, Darbar D, et al. 2012 ACCF/AHA/HRS focused update of the 2008 guidelines for device-based therapy of cardiac rhythm abnormalities. J Am Coll Cardiol 2012;60:1297–313.
13. Curtis AB, Worley SJ, Adamson PD, et al. Biventricular pacing for atrioventricular block and systolic dysfunction. N Engl J Med 2013;368:1585–93.
14. Soteriades ES, Evans JC, Larson MG, et al. Incidence and prognosis of syncope. N Engl J Med 2002;19:878–85.
15. Sra JS, Jazayeri MR, Avitall B, et al. Comparison of cardiac pacing with drug therapy in the treatment of neurocardiogenic (vasovagal) syncope with bradycardia or asystole. N Engl J Med 1993;328:1085–90.
16. Connolly SJ, Sheldon R, Thorpe KE, et al. Pacemaker therapy for prevention of syncope in patients with recurrent severe vasovagal syncope: second vasovagal pacemaker study (VPS II): a randomized trial. JAMA 2003;289:2224–9.

17. Mirowski M, Mower MM, Staewen WS, et al. Standby automatic defibrillator: an approach to prevention of sudden coronary death. Arch Intern Med 1970;126: 158–61.
18. Mirowski M, Morton MM, Reid PR. The automatic implantable defibrillator. Am Heart J 1980;100:1089–92.
19. Mirowski M, Reid PR, Mower MM. Termination of malignant ventricular arrhythmias with an implantable automatic defibrillator in human beings. N Engl J Med 1980;303:322–44.
20. US Food and Drug Administration, 50 Fed Reg 47276, 1985.
21. Connolly SJ, Hallstrom AP, Cappato R, et al. Meta-analysis of the implantable cardioverter defibrillator secondary prevention trials. AVID, CASH and CIDS studies. Eur Heart J 2000;24:2071–8.
22. Moss AJ, Zareba W, Hall WJ, et al. Prophylactic implantation of a defibrillator in patients with myocardial infarction and reduced ejection fraction. N Engl J Med 2002;346:877–83.
23. Coats AJ. MADIT II, the Multi-center Automatic Defibrillator Implantation Trial II (MADIT II) stopped early for mortality reduction, has ICD earned its evidence-based credentials? Int J Cardiol 2002;82:1–5.
24. Bardy GH, Lee KL, Mark DB. Sudden Cardiac Death in Heart Failure Trial (SCD-HeFt) investigators amiodarone or an implantable cardioverter-defibrillator for congestive heart failure. N Engl J Med 2005;352:225–37.
25. Unverferth DV, Magorien RD, Moeschleberger ML, et al. Factors influencing the one-year mortality of dilated cardiomyopathy. Am J Cardiol 1984;54:147–52.
26. Xiao HB, Lee CH, Gibson DG. Effect of left bundle branch block on diastolic function in dilated cardiomyopathy. Br Heart J 1991;66:443–7.
27. Cazeau S, Ritter P, Lazarus A, et al. Multisite pacing for end-stage heart failure, early experiences. Pacing Clin Electrophysiol 1996;19:1748–57.
28. Cazeau S, Leclerco C, Lavergne T, et al. Effects of multisite biventricular pacing in patients with heart failure and intraventricular conduction delay. N Engl J Med 2001;344:873–80.
29. Abraham WT, Fisher WG, Smith AL, et al. Cardiac resynchronization in chronic heart failure. N Engl J Med 2002;346:1845–53.
30. Cleland JG, Daubert JC, Erdmann E, et al. The effect of cardiac resynchronization on morbidity and mortality in heart failure. N Engl J Med 2005;352:1539–49.
31. Bristow MR, Saxon LA, Boehmer J, et al. Cardiac-resynchronization therapy with or without an implantable defibrillator in advanced chronic heart failure. N Engl J Med 2004;350:2140–50.
32. Bilchick KC, Kamath S, Dimarco JP, et al. Bundle-branch block morphology and other predictors of outcome after cardiac resynchronization therapy in Medicare patients. Circulation 2010;122:2022–30.
33. Adelstein EC, Saba S. Usefulness of baseline electrocardiographic QRS complex pattern to predict response to cardiac resynchronization. Am J Cardiol 2009;103: 238–42.
34. Moss AJ, Hall WJ, Cannom DS, et al. Cardiac-resynchronization therapy for the prevention of heart failure events. N Engl J Med 2009;361:1329–38.

Current Status of Transcatheter Aortic Valve Replacement

Kunal Sarkar, MD[a],*, Mrinalini Sarkar, MD[b], Gian Paolo Ussia, MD[a]

KEYWORDS

- Valvular heart disease • Aortic stenosis • Transcatheter aortic valve replacement
- Surgical aortic valve replacement

KEY POINTS

- Aortic stenosis (AS) is the most frequent type of valvular heart disease (VHD) in the West.
- Treatment of patients with AS has been modified with the introduction of transcatheter aortic valve replacement (TAVR).
- Adverse outcomes with first-generation TAVR devices are related stroke, paravalvular regurgitation (PVL), and vascular complications.
- The use of TAVR for treating patients with AS at intermediate or low surgical risk is currently being investigated in large multicenter trials.
- Recognition of severe AS and appropriate referral of patients for TAVR/surgical aortic valve replacement is a cornerstone in altering the natural history of symptomatic AS and ensuring optimal patient outcomes.

INDICATIONS/CONTRAINDICATIONS

The Burden of Aortic Stenosis and Rationale for Transcatheter Aortic Valve Replacement

Degenerative aortic stenosis (AS) is the most common form of valvular heart disease (VHD) encountered in the Western world. The disease process has a long, latent asymptomatic phase.[1] Once symptoms occur, the prognosis of severe AS is dismal, with survival rates of only 15% to 50% at 5 years.[2] The prevalence of AS increases with advancing age and thus is expected to increase with the demographic aging of

Disclosure Statement: G.P. Ussia is a proctor physician for Medtronic Core Valve. Other authors have no disclosures pertaining to this article.
[a] Department of Cardiology, Policlinico Tor Vergata, University of Rome, Tor Vergata, Viale Oxford 81, Rome 00133, Italy; [b] Division of General Internal Medicine, Perelman School of Medicine, University of Pennsylvania, 3400 Spruce Street, Philadelphia, PA 19104, USA
* Corresponding author.
E-mail address: ksarkarmd@gmail.com

world population. The Euro Heart survey examined patients presenting with incident VHD among 92 centers across 25 countries.[3] The mean age of those presenting with valve disease was 65 ± 14 years and AS was the most common form of left-sided native valve disease, occurring in 43.1% of the total patients. In a population-based study from the National Heart, Lung, and Blood Institute database of 11,911 adults across the United States in whom systematic echocardiography was performed, the prevalence of moderate or severe AS was age-dependent from a low of 0.02% in subjects aged 18 to 44 years to a high of 2.8% in patients aged 75 years or older.[4] Surgical aortic valve replacement (SAVR) has been shown to prolong and improve quality of life, even in selected patients over 80 years of age.[5] Nevertheless, many patients do not undergo surgical aortic valve replacement owing to real or perceived increased risks associated with surgery.[6,7]

Transcatheter aortic valve replacement (TAVR) has emerged as an alternative to SAVR in patients who are considered high surgical risk or inoperable due to advanced age and comorbidities. Randomized trials and registry data have demonstrated the safety and efficacy of TAVR in such patients.[8,9] **Box 1** and **Tables 1** and **2** illustrate the indications and contraindications to TAVR in the latest iteration of VHD guidelines issued by the European Society of Cardiology (ESC)[10] and the American College of Cardiology–American Heart Association (ACC-AHA).[11]

Patient Selection and Risk Stratification

The Heart Team approach has received a class I recommendation in both guidelines (ESC and ACC/AHA)[10,11] and is a mandatory requirement for any TAVR program according to the Centers for Medicare and Medicaid Services.

The key functions of the Heart Team include the following (**Fig. 1**).

Determining eligibility and benefit
Evaluation of patients for TAVR is the prime purpose of the Heart Team. Patients are screened and selected for TAVR, SAVR, or medical therapy based on a complex assessment of surgical risk, frailty, concomitant comorbidities, and expectation of meaningful benefit from the procedure. The process seeks to separate patients who are *ill WITH severe AS* from those who are *ill BECAUSE of severe AS*.

Procedural risk assessment
The projection of outcomes after AVR incorporates using risk stratification models. The 2 most commonly used risk stratification algorithms are the Society of Thoracic Surgeons (STS) Predicted Risk of Mortality (PROM)[12] and Logistic European System for Cardiac Operative Risk Evaluation (EuroSCORE) (LES).[13] Both algorithms have been used for selecting patients for TAVR in registries and randomized trials. In general, the LES tends to overestimate mortality in high-risk patients undergoing SAVR and is poorly calibrated for predicting mortality after TAVR. The STS score offers more realistic estimates of postprocedure morbidity and mortality (http://riskcalc.sts.org). An STS mortality score of 8% or higher or a combined morbidity-mortality score of 50% or more is prerequisite for eligibility for TAVR in the United States.

Recently the EuroSCORE II (EUROII),[14] the Aortenklappenregister score,[15] and ACEF (age, creatinine, and left ventricular ejection fraction) model have been developed that allow improved predictive capabilities compared with the LES in patients with TAVR. All current models, including EURO II and STS, are well calibrated for TAVR but were not developed in TAVR populations. A dedicated risk score incorporating frailty, cirrhosis, porcelain aorta, and access approach is likely to greatly improve the ability of the Heart Team in determining risk.

Box 1
Absolute and relative contraindications for transcatheter aortic valve replacement

Absolute contraindications

Absence of a "heart team" and no cardiac surgery on the site

Appropriateness of TAVI as an alternative to AVR, not confirmed by a "heart team"

Clinical

    Estimated life expectancy less than 1 year

    Improvement of quality of life by TAVI unlikely because of comorbidities

    Severe primary associated disease of other valve with major contribution to the patient's symptoms that can be treated only by surgery

Anatomic

    Inadequate annulus size (<18 mm, >29 mm[a])

    Thrombus in the left ventricle

    Active endocarditis

    Elevated risk of coronary ostium obstruction (asymmetric valve calcification, short distance between annulus and coronary ostium, small aortic sinuses)

    Plaques with mobile thrombi in the ascending aorta or arch

    For transfemoral/subclavian approach: inadequate vascular access (vessel size, calcification, tortuosity)

Relative contraindications

Bicuspid or noncalcified valves

Untreated coronary artery disease requiring revascularization

Hemodynamic instability

LVEF less than 20%

For the transapical approach: severe pulmonary disease, LV apex not accessible

Abbreviations: AVR, aortic valve replacement; LV, left ventricle; LVEF, left ventricular ejection fraction; TAVI, transcatheter aortic valve implantation.
  [a] Contraindication when using the current devices.
  Adapted from The Joint Task Force on the Management of Valvular Heart Disease of the European Society of Cardiology (ESC), the European Association for Cardio-Thoracic Surgery (EACTS), Vahanian A, et al. Guidelines on the management of valvular heart disease (version 2012). Eur Heart J 2012;33(19):2451–96; with permission.

Assessing frailty and specific comorbidities

Frailty is defined as a syndrome of decreased physiologic reserve and resistance to stressors, resulting in cumulative declines across multiple organ systems and increased vulnerability to adverse outcomes.[16] The frail phenotype includes weight loss, weakness, poor endurance, slowness, and low activity level. Frailty occurs in at least 50% of patients referred for TAVR and influences mortality.[17] **Tables 3** and **4** enumerate tests for frailty assessment and other specific comorbidities that impact patient selection for TAVR.

Operative approach and feasibility

Multiple access routes are feasible for TAVR. The best approach for TAVR in a particular patient is the one that provides the fewest complications. A multimodality imaging

Table 1
Recommendations for the use of TAVR

Recommendations	Class	Level
TAVI should only be undertaken with a multidisciplinary "heart team," including cardiologists and cardiac surgeons and other specialists if necessary.	I	C
TAVI should be performed only in hospitals with cardiac surgery on-site.	I	C
TAVI is indicated in patients with severe symptomatic AS who are not suitable for AVR as assessed by a "heart team" and who are likely to gain improvement in their quality of life and to have a life expectancy of more than 1 y after consideration of their comorbidities.	I	B
TAVI should be considered in high-risk patients with severe symptomatic AS who may still be suitable for surgery, but in whom TAVI is favored by a "heart team" based on the individual risk profile and anatomic suitability.	IIa	B

Abbreviations: AS, aortic stenosis; AVR, aortic valve replacement; TAVI, transcatheter aortic valve implantation; TAVR, transcatheter aortic valve replacement.

Adapted from The Joint Task Force on the Management of Valvular Heart Disease of the European Society of Cardiology (ESC), the European Association for Cardio-Thoracic Surgery (EACTS), Vahanian A, et al. Guidelines on the management of valvular heart disease (version 2012). Eur Heart J 2012;33(19):2451–96; with permission.

approach is used to assess feasibility for TAVR, select optimal access route, select optimal prosthesis size and type (balloon expandable vs self-expandable), and procedural planning (**Fig. 2**). The components of multimodality imaging and their role in pre-implant assessment are delineated in **Table 5**.

Table 2
Recommendations for treatment of AS: choice of SAVR or TAVR

Recommendations	COR	LOE
Surgical AVR is recommended in patients who meet an indication for AVR (Section 3.2.3) with low or intermediate surgical risk	I	A
For patients in whom TAVR or high-risk surgical AVR is being considered, members of a heart valve team should collaborate to provide optimal patient care	I	C
TAVR is recommended in patients who meet an indication for AVR for AS who have a prohibitive surgical risk and a predicted post-TAVR survival >12 mo	I	B
TAVR is a reasonable alternative to surgical AVR in patients who meet an indication for AVR (Section 3.2.3) and who have high surgical risk (Section 2.5)	IIa	B
Percutaneous aortic balloon dilation may be considered as a bridge to surgical or transcatheter AVR in severely symptomatic patients with severe AS	IIb	C
TAVR is not recommended in patients in whom existing comorbidities would preclude the expected benefit from correction of AS	III: No Benefit	B

Abbreviations: AS, aortic stenosis; AVR, aortic valve replacement; COR, Class of Recommendation; LOE, Level of Evidence; N/A, not applicable; SAVR, surgical aortic valve replacement; TAVR, transcatheter aortic valve replacement.

Adapted from Nishimura RA, Otto CM, Bonow RO, et al. 2014 AHA/ACC guideline for the management of patients with valvular heart disease: a report of the American College of Cardiology/American Heart Association Task Force on Practice Guidelines. J Am Coll Cardiol 2014;63(22):e57–185; with permission.

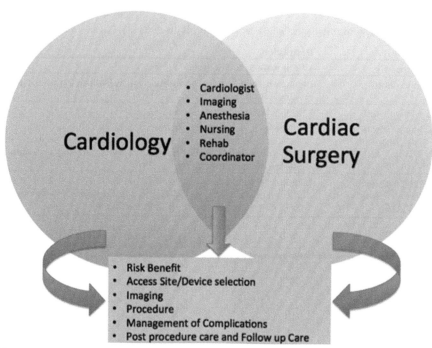

Fig. 1. Components and functions of a TAVR heart team. (*Adapted from* Holmes DR, Mohr F, Hamm CW, et al. Venn diagrams in cardiovascular disease: the Heart Team concept. Eur Heart J 2014;35(2):68.)

Table 3	
Specific comorbidities influencing patient selection for TAVR	
Comorbidity	**Relevance to Selection for TAVR**
CKD	Presence of CKD predicts worse outcome after TAVR.[29] Preprocedural creatinine >1.58 mg/dL is associated with six fold increased risk of mortality.[30]
Coronary artery disease	Presence indicates more extensive vascular disease.[31] Need for staged or concomitant revascularization needs to be assessed. The ongoing ACTIVATION trial is evaluating the role of PCI in TAVR patients.[32]
Mitral valve disease	Up to one-third of patients evaluated for TAVR have severe MVD.[33] Presence indicates more extensive CVD limiting TAVR effectiveness.
Systolic dysfunction	TAVR is generally safe and efficacious. More adverse events but similar overall mortality. Marked improvements in LVEF have been reported after TAVR at 30 d.[34,35]
CLD	Present in 20%–30% of TAVR patients.[36,37] Improved survival and functional capacity compared with medical therapy. Frail patients may not benefit from TAVR in presence of CLD.[38]

Abbreviations: CKD, chronic kidney disease; CLD, chronic lung disease; CVD, cardiovascular disease; LVEF, left ventricular ejection fraction; MVD, mitral valve disease; PCI, percutaneous coronary intervention; TAVR, transcatheter aortic valve replacement.

Table 4
Frailty assessment for patients being evaluated for transcatheter aortic valve replacement

Frailty Test	Description
Gait speed	>7 s to walk 5 m abnormal.
Grip strength	Dynamometer; <30 kg in nonobese man and <18 kg in nonobese woman is abnormal.
6-min walk test	<128.5 m during 6-min walk test.
Comprehensive Assessment of Frailty (CAF)	Grip strength, gait speed, instrumental activities of daily living questionnaire, standing balance test, serum albumin, brain natriuretic peptide, and creatinine. Proprietary scoring algorithm used to measure frailty.
Multidimensional Geriatric Assessment (MGA)	Mini-mental state examination, timed get up and go test, basic and instrumental activities of daily living questionnaires. Frailty index score generated and score ≥ 3 indicated frailty.

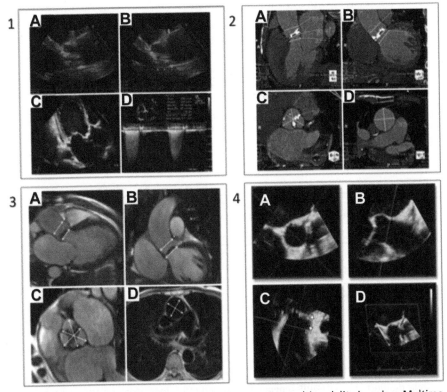

Fig. 2. Assessment of aortic annulus and aortic root using multimodality imaging. Multimodality imaging for TAVR - (1) Assessment of Aortic Stenosis with 2D Echocardiography, (2–4) Pre TAVR assessment of aortic root structures using CT Angiography, Magnetic Resonance Angiography and 3D TEE respectively. (From Tamborini G, Fusini L, Gripari P, et al. Feasibility and accuracy of 3DTEE versus CT for the evaluation of aortic valve annulus to left main ostium distance before transcatheter aortic valve implantation. JACC Cardiovasc Imaging 2012;5(6):579–88, with permission; and Jabbour A, Ismail TF, Moat N, et al. Multimodality imaging in transcatheter aortic valve implantation and post-procedural aortic regurgitation. J Am Coll Cardiol 2011;58(21):2165–73, with permission.)

Table 5
Imaging modalities and their role in TAVR

Imaging Modality	Role in TAVR Planning
Angiography and cardiac catheterization	Assessment of presence and severity of CAD, severity of AS, projection for valve deployment. Assessment of AR, iliac tortuosity, and diameter.
Echocardiography (TTE, TEE)	Diagnosis of severe AS, annulus measurement and prosthesis sizing (3-dimensional TEE).
MDCT	Mainstay of imaging for vascular anatomy and aortic annular size and prosthesis sizing. (Compared to TTE/TEE, MDCT may result in >38% difference in the valve size selected thereby reducing paravalvular regurgitation.) Assessment and measurement of porcelain aorta, coronary artery height, Sinus of Valsalva width, LVOT diameter and calcification, sinotubular and ascending aortic anatomy, and feasibility of a direct aortic approach.

Abbreviations: AS, aortic stenosis; CAD, coronary artery disease; LVOT, left ventricular outflow tract; MDCT, multidetector computed tomography; TAVR, transcatheter aortic valve replacement; TEE, transesophageal echo; TTE, transthoracic echocardiography.

Minimum arterial dimensions required for TAVR are illustrated in **Table 6**.

Alternative access sites may be necessary in patients with challenging ilio-femoral anatomy (calcifications, tortuosity, occlusion). **Fig. 3** illustrates the device characteristics and aortic measurements taken into consideration before implantation of self-expandable devices.

Current Transcatheter Aortic Valve Replacement Platforms

Current TAVR platforms are either balloon expandable valves (BEV) or nitinol-based self-expandable stent-mounted valves. The first TAVR implant was performed in 2002 by Cribier and colleagues[18] in an inoperable patient with severe AS with an equine pericardium valve sewn inside a frame crimped over a balloon catheter. Subsequent iterations of valve and delivery platforms resulted in the Edwards Sapien, the Sapien XT, and recently the Sapien 3 TAVR systems (Edwards Life sciences Inc, CA). The nitinol-based self-expandable core valve (CRS) device has also undergone multiple improvements to its present day iteration, the "Evolut" variant. Characteristic features of these devices are illustrated in **Figs. 3** and **4**.

Table 6
Minimum arterial dimensions for current transcatheter aortic valve replacement platforms

Valve Size, mm	Edwards Sapien	Sapien XT	CoreValve (CRS)	Sapien 3
20		6.0	n/a	
23[a]	7.0	6.0	6.0	5.5
26	8.0	6.5	6.0	5.5
29	n/a	7.0	6.0	6.0
31	n/a		6.0	n/a

[a] Second-generation *Evolut* can be inserted through an 18-F (outer diameter) sheath. Current CRS requires a 22-F outer diameter sheath.

Patient Evaluation Criteria

Product	CoreValve® Evolut™		CoreValve®	
Size	23 mm	26 mm	29 mm	31 mm
Annulus Diameter	18-20 mm	20-23 mm	23-26 mm	26-29 mm
Annulus Perimeter	56.5-62.8 mm	62.8-72.3 mm	72.3-81.7 mm	81.7-91.1 mm
Ascending Aorta Diameter	≤ 34 mm @ 30 mm from annulus	≤ 40 mm @ 40 mm from annulus	≤ 43 mm @ 40 mm from annulus	≤ 43 mm @ 40 mm from annulus
Sinus of Valsalva Diameter	≥ 25 mm	≥ 27 mm	≥ 29 mm	≥ 29 mm
Sinus of Valsalva Height	≥ 15 mm	≥ 15 mm	≥ 15 mm	≥ 15 mm

Fig. 3. CoreValve (CRS) measurements of aortic root structures correlated with device dimensions for appropriate device selection. (Reproduced with permission of Medtronic, Inc. Copyright © Medtronic 2015.)

IMPLANTATION TECHNIQUE AND APPROACHES
The Transfemoral Approach

The transfemoral approach (TF) is the first access choice in a vast majority of centers. It is the least-invasive route and can be accomplished in general anesthesia or deep sedation in a catheterization laboratory or a hybrid room. **Fig. 5** demonstrates the

	Edwards-Sapien(26mm)	Sapien XT(26mm)	Sapien 3(26mm)
Prosthetic Material	**Stainless Steel**	**Cobalt Chromium**	**Cobalt Chromium**
Valve Tissue	Bovine Pericardium	Bovine Pericardium	Bovine Pericardium
Frame Height(Expanded)	16.1mm	17.2mm	20mm
Frame Height(Crimped)	18.1mm	20.6mm	27mm
Crimped Profile	8.3mm	8.0mm	6.7mm
Frame Shortening(Deployment)	2mm	3.4mm	7.0mm
Delivery Sheath ID unexpanded (F)	22/24-F	-16/18/20-F	14/14/16-F
Valve Sizes (mm)	23/26mm	20/23/26/29mm	23/26/29mm

Annular sizes 18-27mm

Valve Sizes 23mm-29mm

Fig. 4. Iterations of the balloon expandable Edwards platforms. (*Adapted from* Webb JG, Wood DA. Current status of transcatheter aortic valve replacement. J Am Coll Cardiol 2012;60(6):483–92; with permission.)

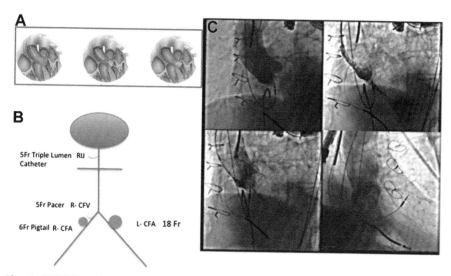

Fig. 5. TF-TAVR: (*A*) concept, (*B*) access sites, (*C*) fluoroscopic demonstration of actual deployment. (*From* Sarkar K, Ussia G, Tamburino C. Core valve embolization: technical challenges and management. Catheter Cardiovasc Interv 2012;79(5):777–82; with permission.)

concept of self-expanding TF-TAVR for core valve (CRS) (**Fig. 5**: 1), basic access sites used for TF-TAVR (**Fig. 5**: 2), and actual valve deployment sequence (**Fig. 5**: 3). **Box 2** describes the sequential steps involved in TF-TAVR. Femoral access was initially obtained with surgical cut down; nonetheless, most centers use a fully percutaneous approach.

Transapical Approach

The transapical approach (TA) was developed for patients with nonoptimal iliofemoral vessels that precluded safe placement of the sheath. For the current iterations of the Edwards Sapien and XT valves, a small anterior minithoracotomy is required for puncturing the apex and inserting a 24 F or larger sheath. With the availability of lower-profile devices for the TF approach, approximately 20% to 30% of TAVR implants using balloon expandable prosthesis are still performed using the TA approach. Potential advantages of the TA route include avoiding diseased and tortuous iliofemoral vasculature, and coaxiality of the prosthesis with the aortic annulus in challenging anatomies. Disadvantages include the need for a thoracotomy, myocardial injury due to apical perforation of the ventricle, and bleeding complications associated with myocardial tears during surgical repair of the apex. **Fig. 6** demonstrates the concept, procedural steps, and fluoroscopic images of valve deployment using a TA approach.[19]

Direct Aortic

The direct aortic (TAo) approach offers the most direct access to the aortic valve. It can be performed either with a mini-sternotomy with a curved J incision in the third intercostal space or a right anterior mini thoracotomy in the second intercostal space.

Box 2
Transfemoral (TF) transcatheter aortic valve replacement (TAVR): procedural steps

- Access. A 6-F to 7-F introducer is used to access femoral artery that is upsized to an 18-F to 22-F introducer sheath
- The native stenotic aortic valve is crossed with a diagnostic Amplatz Left (AL-1) catheter and straight tip wire
- A Super Stiff Amplatz (SSA-1 wire) with a hand-shaped pigtail loop at the end is placed in the LV apex in stable position using the right anterior oblique projection.
- A preimplantation balloon aortic valvuloplasty is routinely performed under rapid right-ventricular pacing with an undersized balloon (1–2 mm smaller than the measured aortic annulus diameter) for preparing the native annulus in all cases except pure aortic regurgitation or degenerated aortic bioprosthesis.
- A pigtail catheter is positioned in the noncoronary cusp as a marker for the annular plane and for contrast injections during the valve deployment. The image intensifier is positioned at the implant angle defined as the optimal left anterior oblique (LAO) projection for aligning the nadir of all 3 coronary cusps in a straight line. The valve is positioned across the aortic annulus and deployed under rapid pacing (Edwards).
- For self-expandable core valve (CRS) deployment, the delivery catheter system (DCS) is positioned such that the horizontal markers of the device are positioned (4–6 mm) below the level of the pigtail catheter (CRS).
- The DCS is maintained as perpendicular to the annular plane as possible and the release is initiated under fluoroscopic and angiographic guidance with repeated small contrast injections (10 mL to 10 mL/s at 900 psi) through the pigtail catheter

---

The TAo approach:

- Avoids a thoracotomy that potentially impedes pulmonary function, especially in patients with chronic obstructive pulmonary disease
- Avoids injury to the myocardium and apex, preserving function in patients with low left ventricular ejection fraction
- Has much less movement on the aorta than TA on the apex, and makes sheath placement easier and safer
- It is compatible with both Sapien and CRS systems
- Direct visualization of the aorta permits rapid cannulation and initiation of cardio-pulmonary bypass for support.

However, the difficulty of crossing the valve in a retrograde direction persists and significant ascending aortic calcification may be a contraindication. The TAo zone is located at approximately the greater curvature of the distal ascending aorta, proximal to the brachiocephalic artery. **Fig. 7** illustrates the procedural steps involved in direct aortic TAVR. **Box 3** enumerates the sequential steps of TAo-TAVR.

Subclavian/Distal Axillary

The trans subclavian approach to TAVR has been successfully used for TAVR since 2006. In a recent study, 2-year propensity-matched outcomes of 141 TAx (transaxillary) versus 141 TF patients found similar rates of procedural success, vascular complications, and survival (74.0% TAx vs 73.7% TF, $P = .78$). Subclavian access

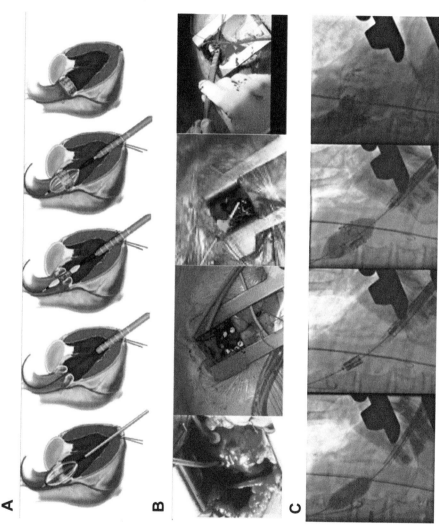

Fig. 6. Transapical (TA-TAVR): (*A*) concept, (*B*) access and closure, (*C*) valve deployment. (*Adapted from* Cheung A, Lichtenstein KM. Illustrated techniques for transapical aortic valve implantation. Ann Cardiothorac Surg 2012;1(2):231–9.)

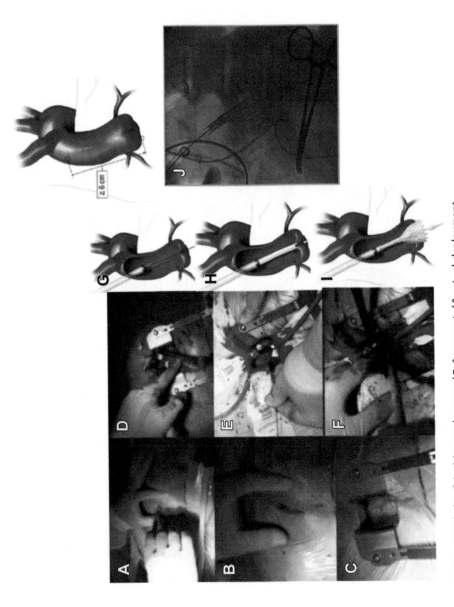

Fig. 7. Direct aortic (TAo-TAVR): (*A–F*) incision and access, (*G–I*) concept, (*J*) actual deployment.

Box 3
Direct aortic (TAo) TAVR: procedural steps

Preprocedure

- Multidetector computed tomography (MDCT) scan is essential to guide in the selection of the
  - Thoracic access location
    - Delivery trajectory should optimize coaxial alignment with native valve and avoid critical vessels
  - Aortic access site
    - Site should be free of calcification and more than 6 cm from the basal plane to facilitate valve deployment
  - The TAo procedure must be performed in a hybrid room that supports both interventional and surgical procedures (eg, Hybrid Operating room)

Procedure (valve deployment)

- Perform aortography with forceps placed directly on the intended access site and use graduated pigtail to confirm ≥6 cm distance from the basal plane
- Place 2 standard double purse-string sutures and gain arterial access via the Seldinger technique or direct cannulation via scalpel puncture
- Maintain the recommended introducer position throughout the procedure to avoid "pop-out" or interaction with the aortic root anatomy
- Position control may be accomplished by the following:
  - Securing introducer with sutures
  - Tunneling the introducer through a skin incision
  - Dedicated hand or operator to manually hold introducer in place
- Perform a standard balloon valvuloplasty
- The TAo procedure provides direct DCS response due to the short and straight approach to the native aortic valve
- Full valve function and partial repositionability before final release provides time for evaluation and adjustment

Procedure (Access Closure)

- Carefully manage purse-string sutures to maintain effective hemostasis during introducer removal
- Consider fast pacing (120–140 beats per minute) or pharmacologic agent to reduce systolic blood pressure below 100 mm Hg

---

should not be considered in a patient with diameter less than 7 mm, significant tortuosity, or previous coronary artery bypass grafting and patent in situ internal mammary artery grafts.[20] The authors have recently described a distal axillary approach to transcatheter aortic valve implantation (TAVI) that is safer and more operator friendly for performing TAVR.[21] **Box 4** and **Fig. 8** illustrate the procedural and technical expedients involved in performing TAVR from a distal axillary approach.

Box 4
Distal axillary access TAVR: procedural steps

Procedure of performing TAVR through distal axillary access

- The left arm of the patient is abducted and externally rotated to 90° for adequate artery exposure. Using an ultrasound probe (linear high-frequency >10 MHz), the axillary artery, axillary veins, and nerves are identified.

- Anesthesia at site of vascular access is administered through the injection of local anesthetic at the level of neurovascular sheath with a 18-G needle. Once the needle reaches the neurovascular sheath, naropin 7.5 mg/mL in 10 mL of physiologic solution (PS) and carbocaine 1% in 10 mL of PS are injected accomplishing a block of the 4 nerves of the axillary plexus (radial, ulnar, median, and the musculocutaneous nerves) under ultrasound guidance.

- The right radial artery is accessed with a 5-F hydrophilic sheath and a 5-F pigtail catheter advanced to the level of the aortic cusps. The right femoral vein is also accessed with a 5-F sheath and a temporary pacing wire was advanced to the right-ventricular apex. The course of the axillary artery is identified and marked on the skin while maintaining the left arm abducted and externally rotated at 90°.

- The surgical technique for exposure of the axillary artery consists of a skin and deep-tissue incision along a line that follows the course of the artery originating from the apex of the axilla and projecting itself into the crook of the elbow. Hence, the median nerve has to be displaced medially and the axillary artery exposed upstream and downstream to the puncture site.

- After isolation, the artery is accessed with an 18-G needle and a 7-F introducer is advanced over a 0.035-inch 145-cm standard guide wire. A 6-F pigtail catheter is positioned in the ascending aorta above the aortic valve plane and the standard guide wire is exchanged for Super Stiff Amplatz wire (Boston Scientific Corp). A small transverse nick is made in the wall of the axillary artery and an 18-F introducer (Cook, Bloomington, IN) is advanced until the distal radiopaque marker is protruding at least 10 mm in the aortic arch. The proximal part of the introducer, at the back-bleed valve level, is secured to the skin with a 00 silk suture to avoid undesired back-and-forth movements.

- The valve crossing and TAVR are performed using the same approach as a TF-TAVR.

- After deployment, the 18-F dilator is reintroduced in the sheath and the entire introducer-dilator assembly is gently removed. Two vascular clamps are positioned upstream and downstream of the access site, respectively, and the incision closed with Prolene 5-0 suture. Finally, a Redon drainage is placed in the surgical wound for approximately 48 hours.

OUTCOMES WITH CURRENT TRANSCATHETER AORTIC VALVE REPLACEMENT PLATFORMS
Clinical Outcomes with Self-Expandable Core Valve

Table 7 highlights important clinical outcomes from large multicenter registries of TAVR with the CRS prosthesis. These studies concur that CRS implantation can be performed with a high procedural success rate (>95%) and excellent 30-day (~90%), 1-year (77%–87%), and 2-year survival (~75%). The ADVANCE registry represents the most contemporary real-world experience with CRS.[22] A total of 44 experienced centers enrolled 1015 patients in this study. The procedural success rate was 97.8% and valve-related complications were extremely low, occurring in fewer than 0.5% of cases. At 30 days, the stroke rate was 2.9%. Major vascular complications occurred in 10.7% and the rate of new pacemaker implantation was

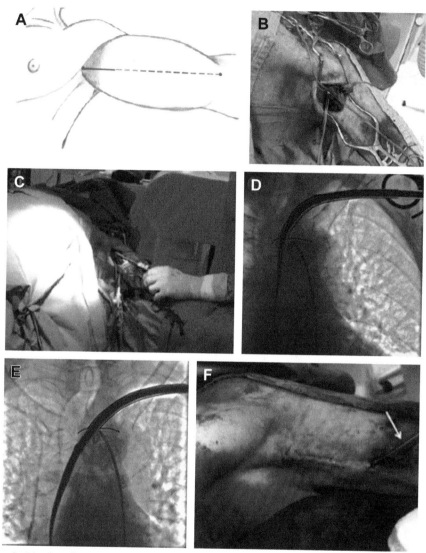

Fig. 8. Distal axillary TAVI: (*A*) concept, (*B*) incision and exposure of distal axillary artery (*C*) placement of 18F introducer, (*D, E*) placement of introducer with tip in the aorta at least 10mm distal to origin of subclavian artery (*F*) closure. (*From* Ussia GP, Cammalleri V, Marchetti AA, et al. Transcatheter aortic valve implantation through distal axillary artery: novel option for vascular access. J Cardiovasc Med (Hagerstown) 2015;16(4):271–8; with permission.)

26.5%. At 12 months, all-cause mortality was 17.9% and cardiovascular mortality was 11.8%.

A major limitation in these registries has been the absence of a core laboratory adjudicating the rates of aortic regurgitation after TAVR. These and other limitations associated with registry data were addressed in the randomized CoreValve pivotal trial.

Table 7
Large transcatheter aortic valve replacement registries with self-expanding prosthesis (CoreValve)

Registry	Total Patients, n	Participating Centers, n	Age of Patients	Logistic EuroSCORE	Procedural Success, %	30-d Stroke Rate	Major Vascular Complications	Permanent Pacemaker, %	30-d Survival, %	1-y Survival, %	2-y Survival, %
Italian[39]	1334	14	82 ± 6	23 ± 15	96.0	1.4[a]	3.3	18.7	88.8	76.4	65.2[b]
FRANCE II[40]	1043	30	82 ± 7	21 ± 14	97.6	4.3[c]	4.5	24.2	90.6	76.3	
UK[36]	1247	25	82 ± 6	19.5	98.2	4.0		24.4	94.2	78.3	76.1
Australia[41]	540	10	84 ± 6	17 ± 11	98.2	3.5	4.1	28.6	96.3	88.0	77.9
Belgian[42]	408	12	82 ± 7	24 ± 15	98.0	4.0		29.0	91.0	80.0	80.0
ADVANCE[22]	1015	44	81 ± 6	19 ± 12	97.8	2.9	10.7	26.3	95.5	87.4	82.1

[a] In-hospital stroke rate reported.
[b] Three-year data.
[c] One-year stroke rate.

CoreValve pivotal trial

The study consisted of 2 arms (**Fig. 9**). The Extreme Risk group was a nonrandomized evaluation of core valve in 471 patients with AS who were at extreme risk for SAVR (ie, >50% chance of mortality or irreversible morbidity) (STS-PROM, 10.3% ± 5.6%; 92% with New York Heart Association class III or IV symptoms).

Major findings of the CoreValve extreme risk study A total of 41 sites in the United States recruited 506 patients, of whom 489 underwent attempted treatment with the CRS.[23]

1. The rate of all-cause mortality or major stroke at 12 months was 26.0% (upper 2-sided 95% confidence bound: 29.9%) versus 43.0% with the objective performance goal ($P<.0001$).
2. Individual 30-day and 12-month events included all-cause mortality (8.4% and 24.3%, respectively) and major stroke (2.3% and 4.3%, respectively).
3. Procedural events at 30 days included life-threatening/disabling bleeding (12.7%), major vascular complications (8.2%), and need for permanent pacemaker placement (21.6%).
4. The frequency of moderate or severe paravalvular regurgitation (PVL) was lower 12 months after self-expanding TAVR (4.2%) than at discharge (10.7%; $P = .004$ for paired analysis).

The randomized arm of the pivotal trial (high-risk study) comparing SAVR with TAVR with CRS was recently published.[9] The following conclusions were drawn from the study.

Major findings of the core valve high-risk study

1. All-cause mortality at 1 year was significantly lower in the TAVR group compared with the surgical group (14.25 vs 19.11%).
2. In this patient population, TAVR was demonstrated to have an absolute risk reduction of 4.9% when compared with surgical AVR ($P<.001$ for inferiority and $P = .04$ for superiority).
3. The results were similar in the intention-to-treat analysis; the event rate was 13.9% for TAVR and 18.7% for surgical valve replacement.
4. There was no significant difference in the stroke rate between the 2 groups.
5. TAVR was shown to be noninferior in terms of echocardiographic indexes of valve stenosis, functional status, and quality of life.
6. The rates of moderate or severe PVL were higher in the TAVR group; however, most of these patients (76.2%) had mild or no regurgitation at 1 year.
7. Surgery had a significantly higher incidence of new-onset or worsening atrial fibrillation, acute kidney injury, and major bleeding.

Clinical Outcomes with Balloon Expandable Prosthesis

Outcomes from large registries of TAVR with BEV are shown in **Table 8**. The results are consistent in underlining that TAVR with BEV is associated with good procedural outcomes (>95%) and 1-year survival (>70%) and acceptable vascular complication and pacemaker implantation rate (<15%).

Placement of Aortic Transcatheter Valve study

The 1-year, 2-year, and 3-year results of the Placement of Aortic Transcatheter Valve (PARTNER) trial (**Fig. 10**), the first multicenter randomized trial comparing TAVR with medical therapy (cohort B) and SAVR (cohort A) with the Edwards Sapien valve in patients deemed inoperable or high risk for SAVR, have been published.

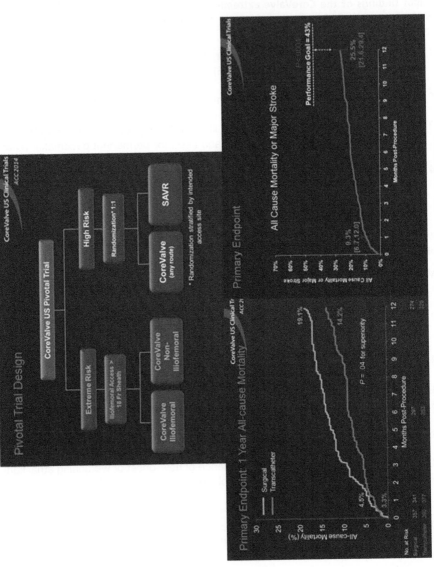

Fig. 9. Core valve trial design and outcomes. (*Data from* Popma JJ, TCT 2013 and Adams DH, ACC 2014.)

Table 8
Large transcatheter aortic valve replacement registries with balloon expandable prosthesis (Edwards)

Registry	Total Patients Balloon Expandable, n	Participating Centers, n	Age of Patients, y	Logistic EuroSCORE, Mean ± SD/Median (IQR)	Procedural Success, %	30-d Stroke Rate, %	Major Vascular Complications, %	Permanent Pacemaker, %	30-d Survival, %	1-y Survival, %
Belgian	187	12	82 ± 7	30 ± 16	97.0	5.0	0.5	5.0	88.0	73.0
Canadian	339		81 ± 8	27.7 ± 16.3	93.3	1.2	13.0	4.9	90.0	76.0
FRANCE	166	30	83 ± 7	25.6 ± 11.4	98.3		11.8	11.8	87.0	NA
FRANCE-2	2107	30	83 ± 7	22.2 ± 14.3	97.0	1.2	7.3	15.6	92.0	76.0
PARTNER-EU	130	9	82 ± 6	30.0 ± 13.7	95.7	2.3	10.8	2.3	86.2	63.1
SOURCE	1038	36	82 ± 7	25.7 ± 14.5	93.8	2.5	7.0	7.0	92.0	76.1
SOURCE-XT	2681	104	82 ± 7	27.0 ± 12.7		2.3	7.3	8.0	93.0	81.0
UK TAVI	410	25	82 ± 7	18.5	97.2	4.1	6.3	7.4	93.0	78.6

Abbreviation: IQR, interquartile range.

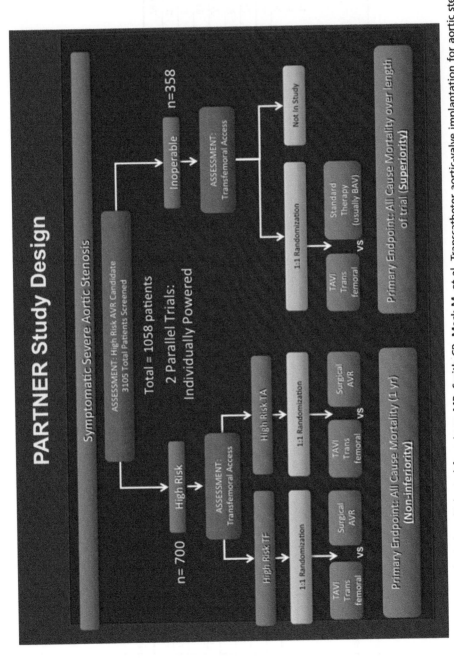

Fig. 10. PARTNER trial study design. (*Adapted from* Leon MB, Smith CR, Mack M, et al. Transcatheter aortic-valve implantation for aortic stenosis in patients who cannot undergo surgery. N Engl J Med 2010;363(17):1597–607.)

Major findings in PARTNER cohort B

1. TAVR-treated patients had a sustained lower 3-year mortality rate than those treated with medical therapy alone (54.1% vs 80.9%, $P<.001$), number needed to treat: 3.7.
2. Those with STS score of 15 or higher had no benefit with TAVR over medical therapy.
3. At 3 years, stroke rate was higher in TAVR (15.7% vs 5.5%, $P = .009$), with a higher proportion of hemorrhagic stroke beyond 30 days, and 6.4% of patients required a pacemaker.

Major findings in PARTNER cohort A

1. Similar 2-year mortality rates were observed with TAVR and SAVR (33.9% vs 35.0%, $P = .31$), with no differences comparing TF with SAVR and TA with SAVR, respectively.
2. The rate of stroke/transient ischemic attack was higher in TAVR (5.5% vs 2.4% at 30 days, $P = .04$, and 11.2% vs 6.5% at 2 years, $P = .05$) but not major stroke alone (4.7% vs 2.4% at 30 days, $P = .10$ and 7.7% vs 4.9% at 2 years, $P = .17$).
3. Major bleeding and vascular complications were predictors of decreased survival. However, a higher than 50% 3-year mortality among inoperable patients serves as a caution for the long-term efficacy of this therapy. Stroke and PVL remain a concern, as well as the lack of benefit of TAVR in extremely high-risk patients (eg, STS score $\geq$15%).

Ongoing trials with transcatheter aortic valve replacement

Encouraging results of TAVR in extreme and high-risk surgical patients have led to the evaluation of TAVR in patients at "intermediate or average" surgical risk (STS score 4%–10%). **Fig. 11** presents the *continuum of surgical risk* and correlates the utility of TAVR or lack thereof with increasing risk. SUrgical Replacement and Transcatheter Aortic Valve Implantation (SURTAVI) **(Fig. 12)** and PARTNER II **(Fig. 13)** are ongoing trials that are evaluating the role of TAVR in patients. **Boxes 5** and **6** detail the principal features of study design, devices, and patient enrollment pertaining to SURTAVI and PARTNER II respectively.

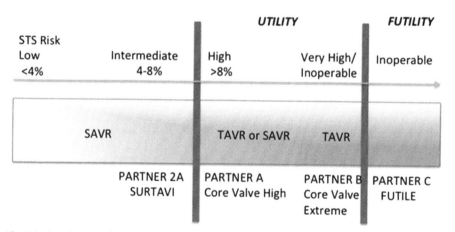

Fig. 11. Continuum of surgical risk and role of TAVR. PARTNER II and SURTAVI trials are evaluating TAVR in patients at "normal surgical" risk (STS >4%). Partner C refers to patients in whom TAVR is futile.

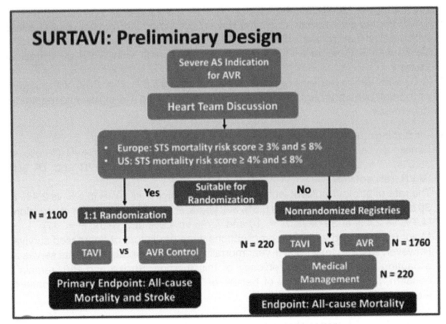

Fig. 12. SURTAVI trial design. (*Adapted from* Serruys PW, TCT 2010.)

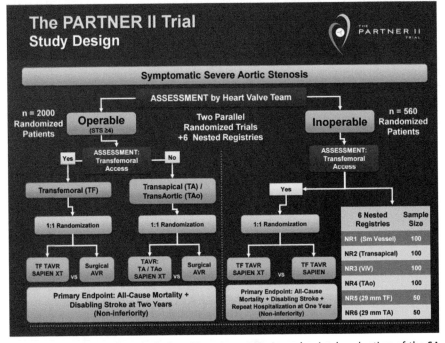

Fig. 13. PARTNER II trial study design. (*From* Leon MB. A randomized evaluation of the SA-PIEN XT transcatheter valve system in patients with aortic stenosis who are not candidates for surgery: PARTNER 2, cohort B outcomes. Presented at: American College of Cardiology Annual Scientific Session; March 10, 2013; San Francisco, CA.)

Box 5
SURTAVI trial design

- The multicenter SUrgical Replacement and Transcatheter Aortic Valve Implantation (SURTAVI) is a 1:1 randomized, noninferiority study comparing CRS with surgical aortic valve replacement (SAVR) across 75 centers in Europe, Canada, and the United States.
- Approximately 2500 patients will be enrolled based on an intermediate Society of Thoracic Surgeons (STS) mortality risk score of 4%–10%.
- Randomization is stratified by need for coronary revascularization, and key inclusion criteria include coronary artery disease (CAD) and Syntax score ≤22, where concomitant percutaneous coronary intervention (PCI) + TAVR or coronary artery bypass grafting (CABG) + SAVR will be performed.
- Key exclusion criteria include multivessel CAD with Syntax score greater than 22, Child C liver cirrhosis, LVEF less than 20%, pulmonary hypertension greater than 80 mm Hg, and chronic obstructive pulmonary disease with forced expiratory volume in first less than 750 mL. Frailty assessment is included in patient selection.
- Primary endpoint is all-cause mortality and major stroke at 24 months. Valve sizes of 23 mm, 26 mm, 29 mm, and 31 mm will be deployed via TF, trans-subclavian, and TAo approaches.

Unresolved issues with transcatheter aortic valve replacement Notwithstanding the rapid evolution of TAVR into a frontline therapy for AS, there are a number of issues impacting patient outcomes. **Table 9** provides a brief overview of factors adversely impacting outcomes after TAVI in contemporary studies and the possible approaches to mitigate their adverse impact on clinical outcomes.

Next-generation transcatheter aortic valve replacement platforms Present day TAVR systems suffer from limitations that contribute to adverse outcomes listed previously. These emerge mainly from the following:

1. Lack of control and accuracy in device positioning
2. Lack of retrievability
3. PVL from inadequate sealing
4. Large profile of delivery catheters and devices

Box 6
PARTNER II trial design

PARTNER II study

The PARTNER II trial is currently under way. The study comprises 2 cohorts:

- Cohort A is a noninferiority study and currently randomizes patients with intermediate operative risk (STS ≥4%), with or without CAD, to TAVR via TF, TA or TAo, or SAVR. Those with revascularizable CAD will receive either PCI + TAVR or CABG + SAVR.
- The primary endpoint for cohort A is 2-year all-cause mortality and stroke.
- Cohort B randomizes patients to the newer Sapien XT-*NovaFlex* system or the Food and Drug Administration–approved Sapien-Retroflex 3 system, while creating 3 additional registries for patients who are not suitable candidates for vascular access with the Sapien valve: small vessel (6–7 mm diameter), cohort B-TA (B-TA), and cohort B-transaortic (B-TAo).

Table 9
Unresolved issues with TAVR and approaches to improve outcomes

Outcome Variable	Unresolved Issues	Approaches to Improve Outcome
Stroke	Multifactorial. Procedure-related factors are responsible for early neurologic events. Late events are influenced by patient-related and disease-related factors.[43] A large meta-analysis revealed that TAVR results in a procedural stroke rate of 1.5% and a 30-day stroke/TIA rate of 3.3%. However, **the 30-d mortality in patients with stroke was 25.5%, 3.5 times higher than the overall rate of 8.1%.**[44]	• Preprocedure imaging to identify high-risk patients and tailoring access approach • Improving procedural technique (wire manipulation, balloon sizing for BAV and device, selective use of BAV and postdilatation) • Use of embolic protection devices during procedure • Anticoagulation after procedure
PVL	>50% of patients with TAVR have mild or greater PVL and/or AR up to 2 y after the procedure.[45] **Moderate–severe PVL/AR is associated with increased all-cause and CV mortality and increase in hospital death by 2.4 times.**[46]	• Accurate device sizing and selection • Imaging to identify extent and distribution of calcium in annulus and LVOT • Device improvement (sealing cuffs, repositionable devices)
Conduction disturbances	CHB requiring PPM implantation seen in 5%–18% (~6.5%) patients post-BEV[47] and 12%–50% (~25%) patients post-CRS.[48] **Risk of PPM 3.7 times higher with CRS. Preexisting RBBB is a predictor of CHB and PPM (OR 8.61).** Persistent LBBB post-TAVR associated with lower LVEF and functional status at 1 y.[49]	• Procedural technique • Appropriate device selection • Identification of device landing zone
Vascular complications	**MVCs associated with decreased 30-d and 1-y survival.**[50] Rate of MVC is 2%–13% in contemporary registries.	• Operator experience • Procedural technique • Identification of calcium and tortuosity on imaging • Lower-profile catheters and delivery sheaths

Abbreviations: AR, aortic regurgitation; BAV, balloon aortic valvuloplasty; BEV, balloon expandable valve; CHB, complete heart block; CRS, self-expandable CoreValve; CV, cardiovascular; LBBB, left bundle branch block; LVOT, left ventricular outflow tract; MVC, major vascular complication; OR, odds ratio; PPM, permanent pacemaker; PVL, paravalvular regurgitation; RBBB, right bundle branch block; TAVR, transcatheter aortic valve replacement; TIA, trans ischemic attack.

A number of new TAVR devices that address these limitations are presently in various stages of clinical evaluation (**Fig. 14**). A representative example of a fully retrievable and repositionable valve system (Lotus; Boston Scientific Corp, Natick, MA) is illustrated in **Fig. 15**. Initial data from REPRISE II (REpositionable Percutaneous Replacement of Stenotic Aortic Valve Through Implantation of Lotus Valve System: Evaluation of Safety and Performance) study evaluating the Lotus valve are encouraging[24] with no cases of significant PVL at 1 year and no instance of valve embolization or coronary compromise.

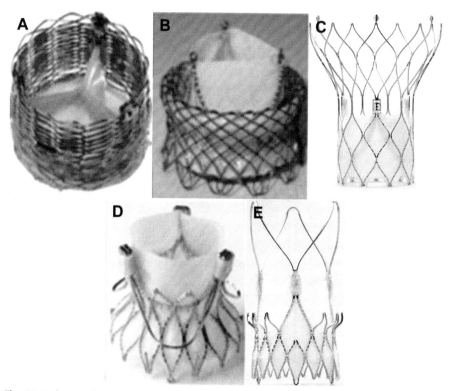

Fig. 14. Valves undergoing early evaluation: (*A*) Lotus (Boston Scientific Corp, Natick, MA), (*B*) HLT (Bracco Inc, Princeton, NJ), (*C*) Portico (St Jude Medical Inc, St Paul, MN), (*D*) Engager (Medtronic Inc, Minneapolis MN), (*E*) Acurate valve (Symetis Inc, Ecublens, Switzerland). ([*A*] Image provided courtesy of Boston Scientific. © 2015 Boston Scientific Corporation or its affiliates. All rights reserved; [*B*] *Courtesy of* HLT, Inc., Maple Grove, MN; with permission; [*C*] Portico and St. Jude Medical are trademarks of St. Jude Medical, Inc., or its related companies. Reprinted with permission of St. Jude Medical, © 2015. All rights reserved; [*D*] Reproduced with permission of Medtronic, Inc. Copyright © Medtronic 2015; [*E*] *Courtesy of* Symetis Inc, Ecublens, Switzerland; with permission.)

Evolving indications for transcatheter aortic valve replacement In addition to the successful use of TAVR to treat degenerated aortic bioprosthesis with severe stenosis/degeneration, other promising areas for further expansion of this technology include treatment of aortic regurgitation and bicuspid valves. The authors published the first successful series of TAVR in severe native AR (Aortic Regurgitation).[25] A recent multicenter registry[26] examined outcomes after TAVR for AR. It demonstrated a lower success rate and increased 30-day and 1-year mortality for patients who underwent TAVR for AR versus AS. Further data from large registries is likely to delineate the role of TAVR in severe native AR.

A number of small studies have reported successful TAVR procedures in bicuspid valves.[27,28] Given the lack of clinical data and anatomic challenges, TAVR for bicuspid valve is still considered on a case-by-case basis.

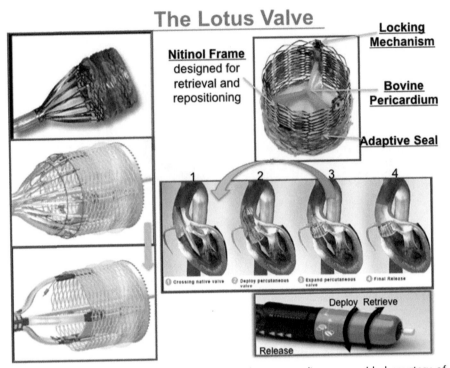

Fig. 15. A fully retrievable and repositionable valve system. (Image provided courtesy of Boston Scientific. © 2015 Boston Scientific Corporation or its affiliates. All rights reserved.)

SUMMARY

TAVR represents one of the most remarkable success stories of interventional techniques applied successfully to a traditionally surgical disease. With rapid improvements in devices and procedure it is anticipated that TAVR will acquire a place of prominence in treatment of aortic valve disease in the not too distant future. Timely referral, appropriate patient selection, evaluation, and procedural planning are key to ensuring excellent patient outcomes with the TAVR approach.

REFERENCES

1. Rosenhek R, Binder T, Porenta G, et al. Predictors of outcome in severe, asymptomatic aortic stenosis. N Engl J Med 2000;343(9):611–7.
2. Carabello BA, Paulus WJ. Aortic stenosis. Lancet 2009;373(9667):956–66.
3. Iung B, Baron G, Butchart EG, et al. A prospective survey of patients with valvular heart disease in Europe: the Euro heart survey on valvular heart disease. Eur Heart J 2003;24(13):1231–43.
4. Nkomo VT, Gardin JM, Skelton TN, et al. Burden of valvular heart diseases: a population-based study. Lancet 2006;368(9540):1005–11.
5. Brown JM, O'Brien SM, Wu C, et al. Isolated aortic valve replacement in North America comprising 108,687 patients in 10 years: changes in risks, valve types, and outcomes in the Society of Thoracic Surgeons National Database. J Thorac Cardiovasc Surg 2009;137(1):82–90.

6. Iung B, Cachier A, Baron G, et al. Decision-making in elderly patients with severe aortic stenosis: why are so many denied surgery? Eur Heart J 2005;26(24): 2714–20.

7. Bach DS, Siao D, Girard SE, et al. Evaluation of patients with severe symptomatic aortic stenosis who do not undergo aortic valve replacement: the potential role of subjectively overestimated operative risk. Circ Cardiovasc Qual Outcomes 2009; 2(6):533–9.

8. Leon MB, Smith CR, Mack M, et al. Transcatheter aortic-valve implantation for aortic stenosis in patients who cannot undergo surgery. N Engl J Med 2010; 363(17):1597–607.

9. Adams DH, Popma JJ, Reardon MJ, et al. Transcatheter aortic-valve replacement with a self-expanding prosthesis. N Engl J Med 2014;371(10):967–8.

10. Authors/Task Force Members, Vahanian A, Alfieri O, et al. Guidelines on the management of valvular heart disease (version 2012): The Joint Task Force on the Management of Valvular Heart Disease of the European Society of Cardiology (ESC) and the European Association for Cardio-Thoracic Surgery (EACTS). Eur Heart J 2012;33(19):2451–96.

11. Nishimura RA, Otto CM, Bonow RO, et al. 2014 AHA/ACC guideline for the management of patients with valvular heart disease. J Am Coll Cardiol 2014;63(22):e57–185.

12. O'Brien SM, Shahian DM, Filardo G, et al. The Society of Thoracic Surgeons 2008 cardiac surgery risk models: part 2–isolated valve surgery. Ann Thorac Surg 2009;88(Suppl 1):S23–42.

13. Nashef SA, Roques F, Michel P, et al. European system for cardiac operative risk evaluation (EuroSCORE). Eur J Cardiothorac Surg 1999;16(1):9–13.

14. Nashef SA, Roques F, Sharples LD, et al. EuroSCORE II. Eur J Cardiothorac Surg 2012;41(4):734–45.

15. Mohr FW, Holzhey D, Möllmann H, et al. The German aortic valve registry: 1-year results from 13 680 patients with aortic valve disease. Eur J Cardiothorac Surg 2014;46(5):808–16.

16. Fried LP, Tangen CM, Walston J, et al. Frailty in older adults: evidence for a phenotype. J Gerontol A Biol Sci Med Sci 2001;56(3):M146–56.

17. Mack M. Frailty and aortic valve disease. J Thorac Cardiovasc Surg 2013; 145(Suppl 3):S7–10.

18. Cribier A, Eltchaninoff H, Bash A, et al. Percutaneous transcatheter implantation of an aortic valve prosthesis for calcific aortic stenosis: first human case description. Circulation 2002;106(24):3006–8.

19. Cheung A, Lichtenstein KM. Illustrated techniques for transapical aortic valve implantation. Ann Cardiothorac Surg 2012;1(2):231–9.

20. Petronio AS, De Carlo M, Bedogni F, et al. 2-year results of corevalve implantation through the subclavian access. J Am Coll Cardiol 2012;60(6):502–7.

21. Ussia GP, Cammalleri V, Marchetti AA, et al. Transcatheter aortic valve implantation through distal axillary artery: novel option for vascular access. J Cardiovasc Med (Hagerstown) 2014;16(4):271–8.

22. Linke A, Wenaweser P, Gerckens U, et al. Treatment of aortic stenosis with a self-expanding transcatheter valve: the International Multi-centre ADVANCE Study. Eur Heart J 2014;35(38):2672–84.

23. Popma JJ, Adams DH, Reardon MJ, et al. Transcatheter aortic valve replacement using a self-expanding bioprosthesis in patients with severe aortic stenosis at extreme risk for surgery. J Am Coll Cardiol 2014;63(19):1972–81.

24. Meredith Am IT, Walters DL, Dumonteil N, et al. Transcatheter aortic valve replacement for severe symptomatic aortic stenosis using a repositionable valve

system: 30-day primary endpoint results from the REPRISE II study. J Am Coll Cardiol 2014;64(13):1339–48.

25. Sarkar K, Sardella G, Romeo F, et al. Transcatheter aortic valve implantation for severe regurgitation in native and degenerated bioprosthetic aortic valves. Catheter Cardiovasc Interv 2013;81(5):864–70.

26. Testa L, Latib A, Rossi ML, et al. CoreValve implantation for severe aortic regurgitation: a multicentre registry. EuroIntervention 2014;10(6):739–45.

27. Wijesinghe N, Ye J, Rodés-Cabau J, et al. Transcatheter aortic valve implantation in patients with bicuspid aortic valve stenosis. JACC Cardiovasc Interv 2010; 3(11):1122–5.

28. Himbert D, Pontnau F, Messika-Zeitoun D, et al. Feasibility and outcomes of transcatheter aortic valve implantation in high-risk patients with stenotic bicuspid aortic valves. Am J Cardiol 2012;110(6):877–83.

29. Thomas M, Schymik G, Walther T, et al. One-year outcomes of cohort 1 in the Edwards SAPIEN Aortic Bioprosthesis European Outcome (SOURCE) registry: the European registry of transcatheter aortic valve implantation using the Edwards SAPIEN valve. Circulation 2011;124(4):425–33.

30. Sinning JM, Ghanem A, Steinhäuser H, et al. Renal function as predictor of mortality in patients after percutaneous transcatheter aortic valve implantation. JACC Cardiovasc Interv 2010;3(11):1141–9.

31. Masson JB, Lee M, Boone RH, et al. Impact of coronary artery disease on outcomes after transcatheter aortic valve implantation. Catheter Cardiovasc Interv 2010;76(2):165–73.

32. Goel SS, Agarwal S, Tuzcu EM, et al. Percutaneous coronary intervention in patients with severe aortic stenosis: implications for transcatheter aortic valve replacement. Circulation 2012;125(8):1005–13.

33. Hutter A, Bleiziffer S, Richter V, et al. Transcatheter aortic valve implantation in patients with concomitant mitral and tricuspid regurgitation. Ann Thorac Surg 2013; 95(1):77–84.

34. Ewe SH, Ajmone Marsan N, Pepi M, et al. Impact of left ventricular systolic function on clinical and echocardiographic outcomes following transcatheter aortic valve implantation for severe aortic stenosis. Am Heart J 2010;160(6): 1113–20.

35. van der Boon RM, Nuis RJ, Van Mieghem NM, et al. Clinical outcome following transcatheter aortic valve implantation in patients with impaired left ventricular systolic function. Catheter Cardiovasc Interv 2012;79(5):702–10.

36. Moat NE, Ludman P, de Belder MA, et al. Long-term outcomes after transcatheter aortic valve implantation in high-risk patients with severe aortic stenosis: the UK TAVI (United Kingdom Transcatheter Aortic Valve Implantation) Registry. J Am Coll Cardiol 2011;58(20):2130–8.

37. Gunter RL, Kilgo P, Guyton RA, et al. Impact of preoperative chronic lung disease on survival after surgical aortic valve replacement. Ann Thorac Surg 2013;96(4): 1322–8.

38. Arnold SV, Spertus JA, Lei Y, et al. How to define a poor outcome after transcatheter aortic valve replacement: conceptual framework and empirical observations from the Placement of Aortic Transcatheter Valve (PARTNER) trial. Circ Cardiovasc Qual Outcomes 2013;6(5):591–7.

39. Barbanti M, Ussia GP, Cannata S, et al. 3-year outcomes of self-expanding Corevalve prosthesis—The Italian Registry. Ann Cardiothorac Surg 2012;1(2):182–4.

40. Gilard M, Eltchaninoff H, Iung B, et al. Registry of transcatheter aortic-valve implantation in high-risk patients. N Engl J Med 2012;366(18):1705–15.

41. Meredith IT, Walton A, Walters D, et al. Mid-term outcomes in patients following transcatheter aortic valve implantation in the corevalve Australia and New Zealand study. Heart Lung Circ 2014;24(3):281–90.
42. Bosmans JM, Kefer J, De Bruyne B, et al. Procedural, 30-day and one year outcome following CoreValve or Edwards transcatheter aortic valve implantation: results of the Belgian national registry. Interact Cardiovasc Thorac Surg 2011; 12(5):762–7.
43. Nombela-Franco L, Webb JG, de Jaegere PP, et al. Timing, predictive factors, and prognostic value of cerebrovascular events in a large cohort of patients undergoing transcatheter aortic valve implantation. Circulation 2012;126(25):3041–53.
44. Eggebrecht H, Schmermund A, Voigtländer T, et al. Risk of stroke after transcatheter aortic valve implantation (TAVI): a meta-analysis of 10,037 published patients. EuroIntervention 2012;8(1):129–38.
45. Kodali SK, Williams MR, Smith CR, et al. Two-year outcomes after transcatheter or surgical aortic-valve replacement. Transcatheter aortic-valve implantation for aortic stenosis in patients who cannot undergo surgery. N Engl J Med 2012; 366(18):1686–95.
46. Abdel-Wahab M, Zahn R, Gerckens U, et al. Predictors of 1-year mortality in patients with aortic regurgitation after transcatheter aortic valve implantation: an analysis from the multicentre German TAVI registry. Heart 2014;100(16):1250–6.
47. Urena M, Mok M, Serra V, et al. Predictive factors and long-term clinical consequences of persistent left bundle branch block following transcatheter aortic valve implantation with a balloon-expandable valve. J Am Coll Cardiol 2012; 60(18):1743–52.
48. Ussia GP, Barbanti M, Petronio AS, et al. Transcatheter aortic valve implantation: 3-year outcomes of self-expanding CoreValve prosthesis. Eur Heart J 2012;33(8): 969–76.
49. Urena M, Webb JG, Tamburino C, et al. Permanent pacemaker implantation following transcatheter aortic valve implantation: impact on late clinical outcomes and left ventricular function. Circulation 2014;129(11):1233–43.
50. Généreux P, Webb JG, Svensson LG, et al. Vascular complications after transcatheter aortic valve replacement: insights from the PARTNER (Placement of AoRTic TraNscathetER Valve) trial. J Am Coll Cardiol 2012;60(12):1043–52.

Chest Pain Evaluation in the Emergency Department

Andrew J. Foy, MD[a], Lisa Filippone, MD[b],*

KEYWORDS

- Chest pain • Myocardial infarction • Acute coronary syndrome

KEY POINTS

- Chest pain is a common chief complaint in the emergency department; approximately 9% of patients with chest pain are diagnosed with an acute coronary syndrome (ACS).
- ACS presents as a range of clinical conditions including unstable angina, non–ST-segment elevation myocardial infarction (MI), ST-segment elevation MI, and sudden cardiac death.
- The patient history and electrocardiogram are very important for early recognition of ACS.
- Type I MI is owing to coronary artery thrombosis, whereas type II MI represents myocardial injury from a variety of underlying processes not related to intracoronary thrombosis.
- Advanced noninvasive testing in patients who rule out for ACS is low yield from a diagnostic standpoint and has not been found to improve patient outcomes.

INTRODUCTION

Chest pain accounts for 5.5 million or approximately 9% of all non–injury-related emergency department (ED) visits for adults in the United States each year.[1] The development of catheter-based therapies and regional care networks allowing for rapid transfer of patients to centers with advanced treatment options has contributed to declining acute coronary syndrome (ACS) case fatality rates. Data from the Nationwide Inpatient Sample shows the overall case fatality in the United States for ST-segment elevation myocardial infarction (STEMI) declined 3% between 1993 and 2009.[2] A community study of patients hospitalized with incident myocardial infarction (MI) in Olmsted County, Minnesota, found the age- and sex-adjusted hazard ratio of death within 30 days for an MI occurring in 2006 compared with 1987 was 0.44.[3]

Despite improvements in the acute care of patients with ACS, it accounts for only a small percentage (9%) of all ED visits for chest pain[4] and there is now concern that current diagnostic strategies could be contributing to the overtreatment of obstructive

[a] Division of Cardiology, Heart and Vascular Institute, Milton S. Hershey Medical Center, Penn State University, 500 University Drive, Hershey, PA 17033, USA; [b] Department of Emergency Medicine, Cooper Medical School of Rowan University, One Cooper Plaza, Camden, NJ 08103, USA
* Corresponding author.
E-mail address: filippone-lisa@cooperhealth.edu

Med Clin N Am 99 (2015) 835–847
http://dx.doi.org/10.1016/j.mcna.2015.02.010
0025-7125/15/$ – see front matter © 2015 Elsevier Inc. All rights reserved.

medical.theclinics.com

coronary artery disease (CAD) in patients presenting with chest pain without evidence of ACS. From 1999 through 2008, the use of advanced medical imaging in patients with chest pain increased 368%.[1] This was largely undertaken in an effort to avoid missing ACS. However, although this strategy has indeed led to the increased detection and treatment of obstructive CAD, it has not translated into a reduction in cardiac events. A cross-sectional, population-based sample of Medicare patients from 1993 to 2001 found that overall hospitalizations for acute MI (AMI) remained flat at 8.7 per 1000 patients despite significant increases in imaging and revascularization rates.[5]

This article discusses the evaluation of patients presenting to the ED with chest pain and suspected ACS. It emphasizes important points of the pathophysiology, patient history, and physical examination, as well as clinical findings related to ACS. It will also discuss recommendations regarding ordering cardiac troponin (cTn) and the use of advanced noninvasive testing in this patient population.

PATHOPHYSIOLOGY

The term 'acute coronary syndrome' refers to any condition that is brought on by a sudden reduction in blood flow to the heart. It represents a spectrum of clinical conditions including unstable angina, non–ST-segment elevation MI (NSTEMI), and STEMI. Unstable angina is characterized by an unstable pattern of ischemic cardiac discomfort without increased cTn levels or ST-segment elevation on the electrocardiogram (ECG). It may or may not present with horizontal or down-sloping ST depression or dynamic T-wave changes on the ECG. NSTEMI is characterized by increased cTn levels. It too may or may not present with evidence of ischemia on the ECG. STEMI is characterized by ST-segment elevation on the ECG owing to transmural (full-thickness) necrosis of the myocardial segment(s) involved. cTn may be negative in the early stage of STEMI because cell lysis and release of intracellular components into the bloodstream do not occur immediately upon myocardial cell death.

AMI is defined by a 20% increase and/or decrease in cTn (I or T), the preferred myocardial biomarker, with 1 value exceeding the 99th percentile upper reference limit (URL) of a normal population.[6] MI can result from a variety of clinical conditions and the etiology of AMI is important to differentiate because it significantly affects patient management. The Third Universal Definition of MI specifies 5 types (**Table 1**).[6] For the purposes of patient evaluation and management, it is best to classify MI into 2 broad categories: (1) MI owing to acute coronary artery thrombosis or (2) MI not owing to acute coronary artery thrombosis, the causes of which are extensive (**Box 1**). The backbone of treatment for patients in the first category is administration of antiplatelet and anticoagulation therapy with or without percutaneous coronary intervention (PCI), which is intended to stabilize the process of acute thrombosis and restore coronary flow. Treatment for patients in the second category is directed at treating the underlying condition responsible for causing oxygen supply/demand imbalance or other myocardial injury (volume resuscitation, presser support, and antibiotics for patients in septic shock).

Coronary artery thrombosis is caused usually by either atherosclerotic plaque rupture or plaque erosion. In each case, there is a loss of integrity in the protective covering over an atherosclerotic plaque, formed by a single layer of endothelial cells, thus exposing the thrombogenic components of the necrotic core to the bloodstream.[7] The resulting intracoronary thrombus is composed of platelet aggregates layered with fibrin, red blood cells, and acute inflammatory cells.[7] Plaque rupture or erosion often occurs at sites without significant luminal stenosis.

One study of 3747 patients in the National Heart, Lung, and Blood Institute Dynamic Registry undergoing PCI found that 216 (5.8%) required additional PCI of the

Table 1 Universal classification of MI	
Type	**Description**
Type 1: Spontaneous MI	Related to atherosclerotic plaque rupture, ulceration, fissuring, erosion, or dissection with resulting intraluminal thrombus; patient may or may not have underlying obstructive CAD.
Type 2: Ischemic imbalance	Oxygen supply cannot meet myocardial oxygen; owing to any condition that affects this relationship including tachycardia, hypotension, severe hypertension with or without LVH, tachyarrhythmias/bradyarrhythmias, anemia, acute bleeding, respiratory failure, or CHF; patient may or may not have underlying obstructive CAD.
Type 3: MI before biomarker evidence of cell death	Symptoms suggestive of AMI and new ischemic ECG changes before biomarker conversion such as in the early phase of STEMI.
Type 4a: Owing to PCI	Troponin rise >5 × 99th percentile URL in patients with normal baseline values (and no concern for AMI before PCI) or a rise of troponin >20% if the baseline values are elevated and are stable or falling.
Type 4b: Stent thrombosis	Evidence of stent thrombosis with an increase and/or decrease of cardiac biomarkers with ≥1 value >99th percentile URL.
Type 5: Owing to CABG	Cardiac biomarker increase >10 × 99th percentile URL in patients with normal baseline values.

Abbreviations: AMI, acute myocardial infarction; CABG, coronary artery bypass grafting; CAD, coronary artery disease; CHF, congestive heart failure; ECG, electrocardiogram; LVH, left ventricular hypertension; MI, myocardial infarction; PCI, percutaneous coronary intervention; STEMI, ST-segment elevation myocardial infarction; URL, upper reference limit.

nontarget lesion within 1 year of follow-up for new clinical symptoms.[8] Although the degree of obstructive CAD during initial PCI was a strong predictor of future events, the majority of new lesions were less than 50% in severity at the time of the initial PCI.[8] The fact that ACS often occurs at sites without significant luminal stenosis is probably 1 explanation for why contemporary PCI trials in patients with stable CAD have not prevented future MI compared with medical management alone.

The "vulnerable plaque" theory identifies several important features of plaque morphology associated with increased odds of rupture and ACS. In 1 study of 1059 patients undergoing coronary CT angiography, the combination of positive remodeling and low-attenuation plaque was associated with a 22% risk of ACS over a mean follow-up of 27 months, whereas 1 feature alone was associated with a 3.7% risk and those with no features a 0.5% risk.[9]

Stable angina is not on the spectrum of ACS and is not considered a medical emergency. Stable angina is most often owing to intracoronary stenosis; however, it can be owing to other processes that compromise coronary flow, such as diastolic dysfunction. Ischemic discomfort follows a stable pattern, often remaining unchanged for months or years at a time, and is caused by the predictable mismatch in myocardial oxygen supply and demand that occurs with exertion and goes away promptly with rest or nitroglycerin. A recent study from a registry of patients with stable CAD found that those with stable angina and evidence of ischemia had a 4% risk of cardiovascular death, MI, or stroke over 2 years of follow-up.[10]

True stable angina is rarely encountered in the ED. In the Internet Tracking Registry of Acute Coronary Syndrome (i*trACS) registry only 1% of chest pain patients were

Box 1
Causes of increased troponin not related to intracoronary thrombosis

Injury related to supply/demand imbalance of myocardial tissue

Tachyarrhythmias/bradyarrhythmias

Aortic dissection or severe aortic valve disease

Hypertrophic cardiomyopathy

Cardiogenic, hypovolemia, or septic shock

Severe respiratory failure

Severe anemia

Hypertension with or without left ventricular hypertension

Coronary spasm

Coronary embolism or vasculitis

Coronary endothelial dysfunction without significant coronary artery disease

Injury not related to myocardial ischemia

Cardiac contusion, surgery, ablation, pacing, or defibrillator shocks

Rhabdomyolysis with cardiac involvement

Myocarditis

Cardiotoxic agents (e.g., anthracyclines, herceptin)

Multifactorial or indeterminate myocardial injury

Heart failure

Stress (Takotsubo) cardiomyopathy

Severe pulmonary embolism or pulmonary hypertension

Sepsis and critically ill patients

Renal failure

Severe acute neurologic diseases (e.g., stroke, subarachnoid)

Hemorrhage

Infiltrative diseases (e.g., amyloidosis, sarcoidosis)

Strenuous exercise

found to have stable angina.[4] Although stable angina is best treated by a cardiologist in the outpatient setting, it is recommended that providers err on the side of caution and consider most cases of characteristic angina in the ED setting as unstable.

In conclusion, ACS presents as a range of clinical conditions caused by a sudden reduction in blood flow to the heart. AMI is defined by myocardial cell death that manifests as a rise or fall of greater than 20% in cTn with at least 1 value exceeding the 99th percentile URL. It is important to determine whether the etiology of AMI is owing to acute intracoronary thrombosis or another cause of myocardial injury, because this information directs appropriate patient management.

PATIENT HISTORY AND PHYSICAL

A thorough history forms the cornerstone of diagnosis for patients who present to the ED with chest pain. In a prospective cohort study of all consecutive patients newly admitted from the ED to 1 academic department of medicine over a 53-day period, researchers found that history alone was the most important modality in patients who were diagnosed correctly based on initial clinical data available on admission.[11]

A high-quality history enables the physician to form a pretest probability of disease. Once this is established, the predictive value of additional findings and tests can be interpreted correctly. Inadequate or inaccurate history taking and failure to appreciate the role pretest probability plays in diagnosing any particular condition exposes the physician to important cognitive biases, which can lead to disproportionate estimates of frequency and faulty Bayesian reasoning.[12]

The differential diagnosis of chest pain is broad. The Internet Tracking Registry of Acute Coronary Syndrome (i*trACS) is a multicenter registry of undifferentiated ED patients with suspected ACS that includes 15,608 patients, with 17,713 visits.[4] Chest pain was the chief complaint in 71% of visits. "Chest pain not otherwise specified" and "other" represented the most common final diagnoses (70%), followed by unstable angina (6.3%), congestive heart failure (4.0%), STEMI (1.6%), pneumonia (1.5%), stable angina (1.2%), NSTEMI (1.0%), pulmonary embolism (PE; 0.4%), pericarditis (0.3%), and dissecting aneurysm (0.1%).

Chest pain characteristics and related symptoms that are associated with increased odds of AMI include pain radiation to both arms (likelihood ratio [LR] 7.1), to the right shoulder (LR, 2.9), to the left arm (LR, 2.3), chest pain as the most important symptom (LR, 2.0), association with diaphoresis (LR, 2.0), and association with nausea or vomiting (LR, 1.9).[13] It should be noted that nausea and vomiting as an isolated symptom(s) is not a predictor of AMI; however, patients with AMI will on rare occasion present with only gastrointestinal complaints. A recent multicenter observational study of 2475 consecutive patients presenting with acute chest pain to the ED found that chest pain aggravated by exertion and chest pain relieved with nitrates also increased the likelihood of AMI.[14] Physical examination findings that are associated with increased odds of AMI include a third heart sound on auscultation (LR, 3.2), hypotension with systolic blood pressure of 80 mm Hg or lower (LR, 3.1), and pulmonary crackles on auscultation (LR, 2.1).[13] Chest pain characteristics that decrease the probability of AMI are pleuritic chest pain (LR, 0.2), pain that is sharp or stabbing (LR, 0.3), pain that is positional (0 LR,.3), and pain reproduced by palpation (LR, 0.2–0.4).[13]

Studies that have examined selected cohorts of ACS patients have consistently found chest pain to be the most common presenting symptom. The population-based MONICA/KORA Myocardial Infarction Registry included 568 women and 1710 men hospitalized with a first-ever AMI.[15] Chest pain or feelings of pressure or tightness in the chest were reported in 93.5% of women and 94.2% of men.[15] An analysis of the Euro Heart Survey, which included 10,253 patients with a discharge diagnosis of ACS, found that the vast majority of patients (>90%) presented with chest pain, either typical or atypical, and this was true regardless of age or gender.[16]

Other studies have found small differences in AMI presentation between men versus woman as well as younger versus older patients. In 1 observational study of 1015 patients younger than 55 years who were hospitalized for ACS, chest pain was the most common symptom in both sexes but women were more likely to present without chest pain than men (19% vs 14%, respectively).[14] An observational study from the National Registry of Myocardial Infarction, 1994 to 2006, that included 1,143,513 patients found women were more likely than men to present without chest pain and so were older versus younger patients.[17] Age was found to be a stronger determinant of different symptoms at AMI presentation than sex.[17] It is also commonly taught that diabetic patients are less likely to present with symptoms of chest pain with ACS; however, there is little evidence to support this. McNulty and colleagues[18] performed coronary balloon occlusion on 100 patients with and without type 2 diabetes and found no difference in the subjective perception of pain between groups; nor were there any differences between men and women.

In summary, chest pain is the hallmark of ACS and specific characteristics of the pain significantly increase or decrease the odds of it. When the patient history is consistent with ischemic cardiac discomfort, physicians should retain a high index of suspicion for ACS despite the lack of objective evidence of ischemia. Finally, although slight differences remain in ACS presentation between men and women physicians should not lose sight of the bigger picture: chest pain is the primary symptom associated with ACS.

CLINICAL FINDINGS
Electrocardiogram

The ECG plays a major role in determining the initial management in patients presenting to the ED with complaints consistent with ACS. The recognition of an STEMI or an "STEMI equivalent" is the first decision point in the management of the patient presenting with an ACS complaint. The 2013 STEMI guidelines refer to a Joint Task Force Definition of MI. It defines diagnostic ST elevation as new elevation measured at the J point of 1 mm or greater ($\geq$0.1 mV) in 2 contiguous leads, in all leads except V2 and V3.[6,19] Given the differences in men and women different levels of elevation are accepted in leads V2 and V3. Abnormal elevation is defined as 2.5 mm or greater in men less than 40 years old, 2 mm or greater in men greater than 40 years old, and 1.5 mm or greater in women.[6]

Three additional ECG patterns deserve special mention in that they may require emergent reperfusion therapy. These are isolated ST depressions in the anterior leads concerning for transmural posterior MI, prominent "hyperacute T waves" in leads consistent with coronary circulation, and isolated ST elevation in aVR with diffuse ST depression. In a 2010 study of approximately 1200 patients looking at the clinical outcomes of patients presenting with isolated anterior segment depression, 26.2% had an occluded culprit artery with increased serum troponin levels.[20] Of these patients, the culprit artery was the left circumflex in 48.4%, the left anterior descending artery in 33.8%, and the right coronary artery in 17.8%.[20] Given the limitation of the standard 12-lead ECG for the evaluation of isolated posterior MI, 3 additional posterior leads (V7, V8, and V9) can be used to aid in diagnosis. In a study of 53 patients undergoing cardiac catheterization, the left circumflex artery was purposely occluded and serial recordings of ST deviation were performed. Compared with the standard 12-lead ECG, the 15-lead ECG was more often able to detect the presence of any ST elevation of 0.5 mm or greater (odds ratio [OR], 2.6) and 1 mm or greater (OR, 2.2).[21]

Patients who present very early after acute occlusion of a coronary artery may not yet display ST segment elevation, but rather prominent T waves, often termed hyperacute T waves.[22,23] This has been described in the literature in human subjects as early as 1934.[24] In a subgroup study of one of the early thrombolytic trials, higher T waves were observed more frequently in patients with a shorter duration of symptoms (2.5 vs 3.3 hours).[25]

Patients who present with an ECG pattern of ST depression and isolated ST elevation in aVR while not meeting the criteria for acute STEMI are frequently managed with an early invasive strategy owing to the concern for left main or severe multivessel disease.[26,27] In a multivariable analysis of NSTEMI patients, 140 of whom met this pattern, those with ST depression and isolated elevation in aVR showed an increased risk of culprit left main disease (OR, 4.7) and in-hospital cardiovascular mortality (OR,

5.6) compared with patients without any ST deviation. Patients with isolated ST depression did not demonstrate this risk. Additionally, at 1-year follow-up, ST depression and isolated ST elevation in aVR was a strong predictor of cardiovascular death (hazard ratio, 2.3).[27]

As mentioned, ST segment depressions can be observed with isolated posterior wall MI and in association with elevation in aVR. ST depressions may also be observed in association with STEMI, termed reciprocal ST change. However, ST segment depression alone may represent subendocardial ischemia. The morphology of ST segment depression that is most consistent with ischemia is horizontal or downsloping. The degree of depression considered significant is 0.5 mm or greater measured at the J point. Both the amount of depression and the extent of depression are associated with an increased risk of death.[28,29] In a 2001 study looking at patients who were enrolled in the PARAGON-A study, patients whose presenting ECG had ST depression of 0.2 mm or greater had an OR of 5.7 for death at 1 year.[30] Additionally, when those depressions involved more than 1 region, their risk of death increased with an OR of 9.2 compared with no ST segment depression.[30]

T wave inversions are encountered commonly in patients presenting with ACS. T wave inversion may present alone or with ST segment depression. Significant T wave inversions are generally 1 mm or greater in depth and occur in 2 or more contiguous leads. The prognostic importance of T wave inversion alone is not clear; however, 2 particular patterns of T wave inversion historically portent a high risk of anterior wall MI. This pattern described by de Zwann and colleagues[31] in 1982 is referred to as Wellens' warning. This pattern of either symmetric deep T wave inversion or a sharply biphasic T wave in the anterior precordial leads is treated with an early invasive strategy. Of note, this pattern often occurs after a chest pain episode and may normalize during recurrent pain episodes.[31–33]

There are many underlying conditions that confound the diagnosis of ACS. The presence of bundle branch blocks, left ventricular hypertrophy, paced rhythms, Brugada syndrome, left ventricular aneurysm, and early repolarization pattern all may have ST segment elevations on the baseline ECG. Similarly, ST depressions may be observed in bundle branch blocks, left ventricular hypertrophy, digitalis effect, and electrolyte abnormalities.

Patients presenting with chest pain that is not ACS often have changes on their EGC. There are many ECG abnormalities described in patients with PE; these abnormalities include S1Q3T3, S1S2S3, right bundle branch block, low voltage, and right axis deviation. Additionally, T wave changes that may mimic ACS have been observed. In a study of 80 patients admitted with PE, 68% had an ischemic T wave pattern on their ECG (85% of patients with massive PE and 19% in nonmassive PE).[34] In a more recent study of 127 patients, 40 diagnosed with PE and 87 diagnosed with ACS, negative T waves were seen in leads III and V1 in 88% of PE patients compared with only 1% of ACS patients.[35]

Patients presenting with chest pain owing to pericarditis may demonstrate several different ECG abnormalities. Classically, there is a progression through 4 stages. The first stage with ST segment elevation can be misinterpreted as STEMI. However, unlike STEMI, ST elevation in pericarditis is usually diffuse. Additionally, there may be PR depression identified most often in lead II.[36] The opposite findings are observed in aVR in patients with pericarditis with PR elevation and ST depression.

Patients with acute aortic dissection often have EGC changes that are consistent with myocardial ischemia or may present with clear ST elevation. In a recent study of 233 patients diagnosed with Stanford type A acute aortic dissection, approximately 50% of patients had ST–T wave changes (4% with ST elevation, 47% with ST depression and/or negative T waves).[37] Patients in this study with ST–T wave changes had a poorer clinical condition and subsequent higher mortality when compared with patients who had normal or no significant ST–T changes on admission.[37]

In conclusion, the ECG is integral in the evaluation of the patient with suspected ACS. The patient's presentation and risk factors for ACS as well as for other non-ACS causes of chest pain should be interpreted in conjunction with the ECG to avoid misdiagnosis.

Cardiac Troponin

cTn is the preferred biomarker for diagnosing AMI because of its superior sensitivity and specificity for detection of myocardial necrosis. It is an important part of the myocardial contractile apparatus and is released into the bloodstream, over time (from 30 minutes to 12 hours) after cardiomyocyte death.[6] AMI is defined by an increase or decrease of greater than 20% in cTn with at least 1 value exceeding the 99th percentile URL. It must be kept in mind that despite the high specificity of cTn for myocardial necrosis, it is not specific for the cause of injury. Maag and colleagues[38] found that in a large, undifferentiated cohort of patients who underwent cTn testing in the ED that when "chest pain" was not the chief complaint, an elevated cTn that met the definition for AMI was unlikely to be owing to type I MI (20%). However, when "chest pain" was the chief complaint, nearly all patients with an elevated cTn had a type I MI (OR, 7.3).[38] Because this is an article on the evaluation of chest pain, we will not belabor this point. It suffices to say that, when chest pain is not the chief complaint, caution should be exercised in ordering cTn and interpreting the result.

Physicians should be aware of the 99th percentile URL for the cTn assay used in their hospital because all cTn assays have different URLs. Ideally, a cTn assay should have a coefficient of variation of less than 10% above the 99th percentile URL. Levels below the 99th percentile URL are often reported. Failure to appreciate this concept could lead physicians to misinterpret normal cTn levels as significant elevations. Therefore, physicians must familiarize themselves with the performance characteristics of the cTn assay used in their laboratories.

Serial measurements of cTn are necessary when cTn concentration is not elevated on admission because cTn may not be detectable in the blood within the first hours after myocardial injury.[39] When myocardial ischemia is suspected and cTn is not initially detected, the current standard of care in the United States calls for a cTn to be drawn again in 6 to 9 hours, although precise timing is not defined. If the index of suspicion is high then a third sample should be drawn in 12 to 24 hours.[39]

IMAGING AND ADDITIONAL TESTING

In 2007, the American College of Cardiology and American Heart Association produced guidelines for the management of patients with unstable angina and NSTEMI. This report was developed in collaboration with the American College of Emergency Physicians, the Society for Cardiovascular Angiography and Interventions, and the Society for Thoracic Surgeons.[39] It was also endorsed formally by the American Association of Cardiovascular and Pulmonary Rehabilitation and the Society for Academic Emergency Medicine. It states that,

> In patients with suspected ACS in whom ischemic heart disease is present or suspected, if the follow-up 12-lead ECG and cardiac biomarkers measurements are normal, a stress test (exercise or pharmacological) to provoke ischemia should be performed in the ED, in a chest pain unit, or on an outpatient basis in a timely

fashion (within 72 h) as an alternative to inpatient admission. Low-risk patients with a negative diagnostic test can be managed as outpatients.

It was given a class I recommendation, meaning the "benefit >>> risk" and "procedure/treatment SHOULD be performed/administered." However, it was also assigned a level C for estimate of certainty of treatment effect, meaning there is little if any evidence to support it outside of expert opinion. This recommendation has not been updated with the exception of a 2010 scientific statement from the American Heart Association, which adds that anatomic assessment, meaning coronary CT angiography, could be performed in place of stress testing.[40]

Despite these recommendations, significant questions remain with the most important being; Does our current practice improve patient outcomes? Several retrospective studies suggest the answer is "no." Chan and colleagues[41] performed a prospective cohort study on 832 consecutive patients who presented to a single ED with chest pain and were admitted to a non–intensive care telemetry bed over a 16-month period. Thirty-one percent of patients received either an inpatient or outpatient stress test in the form of exercise electrocardiography. At baseline, there were no differences between patients who received stress testing or not in respect to demographics, risk factors, risk scores (Acute Coronary Ischemia–Time Insensitive Predictive Instrument [ACI-TIPI] and Goldman), or specific clinical features of the chest pain, including location, quality, or associated symptoms.[41] The authors found that more than 30 days of follow-up the overall rate of AMI among the cohort was low (<1%) and there was no difference between patients who received stress testing and those who did not.[41] Given the low event rate, the authors cautioned that the sample size was too small to exclude a type II error with confidence.[41]

Safavi and colleagues[42] recently performed a cross-sectional study of 224 hospitals using administrative claims data for 549,078 patients with suspected ischemia on initial evaluation. The aim was to characterize hospital variation in use of noninvasive cardiac imaging and the association of imaging use with downstream testing, interventions, and outcomes. They found that imaging rates for hospitals in the highest quartile was 34.8%, whereas the lowest quartile was 6.0%.[42] This large difference in noninvasive imaging was associated with an increase in downstream coronary angiography (Q1, 1.2% vs Q4, 4.9%) and revascularization procedures (Q1, 0.5% vs Q4, 1.9%); however, readmission rates for AMI within 2 months were the same.[42]

Foy and colleagues[43] compared chest pain testing strategies in a national cohort of 421,774 privately insured patients. Individuals were selected who presented to the ED with a primary or secondary diagnosis of chest pain and were classified into 1 of 5 initial testing strategies, which included no noninvasive testing, exercise ECG, stress echocardiography, myocardial perfusion scintigraphy, or coronary CT angiography within 7 days of the index encounter. The main outcome measures included the percentage of patients in each group who received a cardiac catheterization, coronary revascularization procedure, future noninvasive test, or who were hospitalized for AMI over 7 and 190 days of follow-up. The authors found that noninvasive testing was associated with significantly higher odds of catheterization and revascularization, but no difference in hospitalizations for AMI, suggesting that noninvasive testing does not reduce missed MIs.[43] They estimated that for every 27 patients who undergo myocardial perfusion scintigraphy (the most common stress testing strategy) instead of an initial strategy of no testing, 1 will undergo an unnecessary catheterization.[42] For every 166 patients who undergo myocardial perfusion scintigraphy instead of no testing, 1 will undergo an unnecessary revascularization procedure.[43]

The 3 studies challenge the existing American College of Cardiology/American Heart Association (ACC/AHA) recommendations and provide the best evidence that is currently available regarding downstream testing, interventions, and outcomes related to noninvasive testing strategies in this patient population.[41–43] However, all studies were observational in nature and limited by their inability to control for unmeasured confounders. Furthermore, the studies by Safavi and colleagues and Foy and colleagues assess broad populations of patients and are unable to assess for specific clinical characteristics of the chest pain complaint that could influence the utility of noninvasive testing. Perhaps there are subgroups of patients within the broader population of low-risk chest pain patients who benefit from noninvasive testing.

Foy and colleagues[44] hypothesized that the Diamond score would have diagnostic and prognostic utility in patients who present to the ED with chest pain and rule out for ACS. The Diamond score classifies chest pain based on 3 criteria: (1) substernal location (2) brought on by physical exertion or emotional stress and (3) relieved with rest or nitroglycerin? Pain that fulfills 3 of 3 of these criteria is "typical," 2 of 3 is "atypical," and 1 of fewer of the 3 is "nonanginal." In a retrospective study of 502 consecutive ED observation unit patients without a history of CAD who underwent stress echocardiography, 90% had "nonanginal" or "atypical" chest pain.[44] In these patients, the positive predictive value of stress echocardiography was 0% and no patients experienced a 30-day major adverse cardiac event.[44] However, in the 10% of patients with "typical" chest pain, the positive predictive value of stress testing was 75% and 15% underwent revascularization for a presumptive diagnosis of ACS.[44]

Data from these studies were used by Foy and Sciamanna to develop an informed decision making script that was tested in a prospective, randomized clinical vignette study of 176 patients being seen in a general internal medicine office (Foy AJ, Sciamanna C. Special communication, 2014). All participants received an identical question stem, which involved presenting to the ED with chest pain, ruling out for AMI, and being told their pain was "atypical." They were randomized to either a standard recommendation for stress testing based on the ACC/AHA guidelines or informed decision making. Patients in the informed decision making group were given additional information (155 words) that included the following:

> Like all tests, a stress test is not perfect. For every 100 patients like you who have a stress test, about 95 will have normal results. One or two will have an abnormal stress test and get a heart catheterization and either a stent or bypass surgery – which may or may not prevent a future heart attack. Three or four will have an abnormal stress test but a normal heart catheterization, meaning the stress test was inaccurate. Which would you choose? Option 1: Have a stress test in the next 3 days. Option 2: Do nothing now until I see my primary care doctor.

Informed decision making led to a significant reduction in patients desire to undergo stress testing (29.2% vs 90.8%) (Foy AJ, Sciamanna C. Special communication). On multivariate analysis, those who received informed decision making were 97% less likely to choose stress testing (Foy AJ, Sciamanna C. Special communication). Age, gender, education status, tobacco use, and comorbid conditions did not impact patients desire to undergo stress testing. This study suggests that, when presented with accurate information on stress testing in the event of presenting to the ED with low-risk chest pain, a small percentage of patients actually desire it. Given the paucity of data supporting this practice and the significant resources it consumes, we advocate an informed decision-making approach.

FUTURE CONSIDERATIONS/SUMMARY

The practice of chest pain evaluation in the ED continues to evolve. Recently, high-sensitivity cTn assays have shown promise in expediting the disposition of these patients; however, there are concerns regarding specificity.[45] They are not yet available in the United States. In addition, risk score models continue to evolve. The HEART and Diamond scores take into account specific characteristics of the patient history and show potential for accurately predicting patient risk.[44] An optimal strategy would be to pair an expedited rule out ($\leq$2 hours) with a risk score model like the Diamond score to identify a large percentage of patients who are safe for discharge without further noninvasive testing. Such a strategy would streamline significantly the process of evaluation in the ED and save countless resources; however, it would have to be tested in prospective clinical trials and thus its prospects remain distant.

REFERENCES

1. Bhuiya F, Pitts SR, McCaig LF. Emergency department visits for chest pain and abdominal pain: United States, 1999–2008. NCHS data brief, no 43. Hyattsville (MD): National Center for Health Statistics; 2010.
2. Dabhadkar KC, Kulshreshtha A, Deshmukh AJ, et al. National trends in case fatality based on anatomical location of ST elevation myocardial infarction in hospitalized patients, 1993–2009. Circulation 2012;126:A17693.
3. McManus DD, Gore J, Yarzebski J, et al. Recent trends in the incidence, treatment, and outcomes of patients with ST and non-ST-segment acute myocardial infarction. Am J Med 2011;124:40–7.
4. Lindsell CJ, Anantharaman V, Diercks D, et al. The Internet Tracking Registry of Acute Coronary Syndromes (i*trACS): a multicenter registry of patients with suspicion of acute coronary syndromes reported using the standardized reporting guidelines for emergency department chest pain studies. Ann Emerg Med 2006;48:666–77.
5. Lucas FL, DeLorenzo MA, Siewers AE, et al. Temporal trends in the utilization of diagnostic testing and treatments for cardiovascular disease in the United States, 1993–2001. Circulation 2006;113:374–9.
6. Thygesen K, Alpert JS, Jaffe AS, et al, The Writing Group on behalf of the Joint ESC/ACCF/AHA/WHF Task Force for the Universal Definition of Myocardial Infarction. Third universal definition of myocardial infarction. Circulation 2012;126:2020–35.
7. Virmani R, Kolodgie FD, Burke AP, et al. Lessons from sudden coronary death: a comprehensive morphological classification scheme for atherosclerotic lesions. Arterioscler Thromb Vasc Biol 2000;20:1262–75.
8. Glaser R, Selzer F, Faxon DP, et al. Clinical progression of incidental, asymptomatic lesions discovered during culprit vessel coronary intervention. Circulation 2005;111:143–9.
9. Motoyama S, Sarai M, Harigaya H, et al. Computed tomographic angiography characteristics of atherosclerotic plaques subsequently resulting in acute coronary syndrome. J Am Coll Cardiol 2009;54:49–57.
10. Steg PG, Greenlaw N, Tendera M, et al. Prevalence of anginal symptoms and myocardial ischemia and their effect on clinical outcomes in outpatients with stable coronary artery disease. JAMA Intern Med 2014;174:1651–9.
11. Paley L, Zornitzki T, Cohen J, et al. Utility of clinical examination in the diagnosis of emergency department patients admitted to the Department of Medicine of an Academic Hospital. Arch Intern Med 2011;171(15):1394–6.

12. Croskerry P. Achieving quality in clinical decision making: cognitive strategies and detection of bias. Acad Emerg Med 2002;9:1184–204.
13. Panju AA, Hemmelgarn BR, Guyatt GH, et al. The rational clinical examination: is this patient having a myocardial infarction. JAMA 1998;280:1256–63.
14. Gimenez MR, Reiter M, Twerenbold R, et al. Sex-specific chest pain characteristics in the early diagnosis of acute myocardial infarction. JAMA Intern Med 2014;174:241–9.
15. Kirchbeger I, Heier M, Kuch B, et al. Sex differences in patient-reported symptoms associated with myocardial infarction (from the population-based MONICA/KORA myocardial infarction registry). Am J Cardiol 2011;107:1585–9.
16. Rosengren A, Wallentin L, Gitt AK, et al. Sex, age, and clinical presentation of acute coronary syndromes. Eur Heart J 2004;25:663–70.
17. Canto JG, Rogers WJ, Goldberg RJ, et al. Association of age and sex with myocardial infarction symptom presentation and in-hospital mortality. JAMA 2012;307:813–22.
18. McNulty PH, Ettinger SM, Gascho J, et al. Comparison of subjective perception of myocardial ischemia produced by coronary balloon occlusion in patients with versus those without type 2 diabetes mellitus. Am J Cardiol 2003;91:965–8.
19. O'Gara PT, Kushner FG, Ascheim DD, et al. 2013 ACCF/AHA guideline for the management of ST-elevation myocardial infarction. J Am Coll Cardiol 2013;61:485–510.
20. Pride YB, Tung P, Mohanavelu S, et al. Angiographic and clinical outcomes among patients with acute coronary syndromes presenting with isolated anterior ST-segment depression: a TRITON-TIMI 38 (Trial to assess improvement in therapeutic outcomes by optimizing platelet inhibition with prasugrel-thrombolysis in myocardial infarction 38) substudy. JACC Cardiovasc Interv 2010;3:806–11.
21. Aqel RA, Hage FG, Ellipeddi P, et al. Usefulness of three posterior chest leads for the detection of posterior wall acute myocardial infarction. Am J Cardiol 2009;103:159–64.
22. Somers MP, Brady WJ, Perron AD, et al. The prominent T wave: electrocardiographic differential diagnosis. Am J Emerg Med 2002;20:243–51.
23. Sovari AA, Assadi R, Lakshminarayanan B. Hyperacute T wave, the early sign of myocardial infarction. Am J Emerg Med 2007;25:859.e1–7.
24. Wood FC, Wolferth CC. Huge T-waves in precordial leads in cardiac infarction. Am Heart J 1934;9:706–21.
25. Hochrein J, Sun F, Pieper KS, et al. Higher T-wave amplitude associated with better prognosis in patients receiving thrombolytic therapy for acute myocardial infarction (a GUSTO-I Substudy). Am J Cardiol 1998;81:1078–84.
26. Yan AT, Yan RT, Kennelly BM, et al. Relationship of ST elevation in lead aVR with angiographic findings and outcomes in non-ST elevation acute coronary syndromes. Am Heart J 2007;154:71–8.
27. Taglieri N, Marzocchi A, Saia F, et al. Short- and long-term prognostic significance of ST-segment elevation in lead aVR in patients with non-ST-segment elevation acute coronary syndrome. Am J Cardiol 2011;108:21–8.
28. Kaul P, Fu Y, Chang WC, et al. Prognostic value of ST segment depression in acute coronary syndromes: insights from PARAGON-A applied to GUSTO-IIb. J Am Coll Cardiol 2001;38:64–71.
29. Savonitto S, Cohen MG, Politi A, et al. Extent of ST-segment depression and cardiac events in non-ST-segment elevation acute coronary syndromes. Eur Heart J 2005;26:2106–13.
30. The PARAGON Investigators. International, randomized, controlled trial of lamifiban (a platelet plycoprotein IIb/IIIa inhibitor), heparin, or both in unstable angina. Circulation 1998;97:2386–95.

31. de Zwann C, Bar FW, Wellens HJ. Characteristic electrocardiographic pattern indicating a critical stenosis high in left anterior descending coronary artery in patients admitted because of impending myocardial infarction. Am Heart J 1982; 103:730–6.
32. Lilaonikul M, Robinson K, Roberts M. Wellens' syndrome: significance of ECG pattern recognition in the emergency department. Emerg Med J 2009;26:750–1.
33. Agarwal R, Mehrotra AK, Swamy RS. Wellens syndrome: a life-saving diagnosis. Am J Emerg Med 2012;30:255.e3–5.
34. Ferrari E, Imbert A, Chevalier T, et al. The ECG in pulmonary embolism predictive of negative T waves in precordial leads- 80 case reports. Chest 1997;111:537–44.
35. Kosuge M, Kimura K, Ishikawa T, et al. Electrocardiographic differentiation between acute pulmonary embolism and acute coronary syndromes on the basis of negative T waves. Am J Cardiol 2007;99:817–21.
36. Porela P, Kytö V, Nikus K, et al. PR depression is useful in the differential diagnosis of myopericarditis and ST elevation myocardial infarction. Ann Noninvasive Electrocardiol 2012;17:141–5.
37. Kosuge M, Uchida K, Imoto K, et al. Frequency and implication of ST-T abnormalities on hospital admission electrocardiograms in patients with type A acute aortic dissection. Am J Cardiol 2013;112:424–9.
38. Maag R, Sun S, Hannon M, et al. Positive predictive value of an elevated cardiac troponin for type I myocardial infarction in emergency department patients based on the chief complaint. Am J Emerg Med 2015. [Epub ahead of print].
39. Anderson JL, Adams CD, Antman EM, et al. ACC/AHA 2007 guidelines for the management of patients with unstable angina/non-ST-elevation myocardial infarction. J Am Coll Cardiol 2007;50:e1–157.
40. Amsterdam EA, Kirk D, Bluemke DA, et al. Testing of low-risk patients presenting to the emergency department with chest pain: a scientific statement from the American Heart Association. Circulation 2010;122:1756–76.
41. Chan GW, Sites FD, Shofer FS, et al. Impact of stress testing on 30-day cardiovascular outcomes for low-risk patients with chest pain admitted to floor telemetry beds. Am J Emerg Med 2003;21:282–7.
42. Safavi KC, Li S, Dharmarajan K, et al. Hospital variation in the use of noninvasive cardiac imaging and its association with downstream testing, interventions, and outcomes. JAMA Intern Med 2014;174:546–53.
43. Foy AJ, Liu G, Davidson WR, et al. Comparative effectiveness of diagnostic testing strategies in emergency department patients with chest pain: an analysis of downstream testing, interventions, and outcomes. JAMA Intern Med 2015;175: 428–36.
44. Foy AJ, Baquero GA, Naccarelli GV, et al. Applying the diamond criteria could improve utilization of stress echocardiography for patients who present to the emergency department with low-risk chest pain. Crit Pathw Cardiol 2014;13: 49–54.
45. Than M, Cullen L, Reid CM, et al. A 2-h diagnostic protocol to assess patients with chest pain symptoms in the Asia-Pacific region (ASPECT): a prospective observational validation study. Lancet 2011;377:1077–84.

Cardiac MRI

A General Overview with Emphasis on Current Use and Indications

Michael P. Pfeiffer, MD[a], Robert W.W. Biederman, MD, FSGC[b,c,*]

KEYWORDS

- MRI • Cardiac MRI (CMR) • Cardiomyopathy, nonischemic • Ischemic heart disease
- Intracardiac masses

KEY POINTS

- Cardiac MRI (CMR) has both established and evolving uses in cardiovascular imaging.
- CMR is the reference standard in many areas of cardiovascular imaging; however, its routine use is limited by several factors.
- Understanding the basics CMR image acquisition and safety are paramount to appropriate utilization.
- The ordering physician supplies the clinical entity or question for CMR. The CMR protocol is derived by the performing facility.
- CMR should be used or considered in select clinical conditions and whenever more traditional imaging modalities are insufficient or incongruent in their information.

INTRODUCTION

MRI is simultaneously a well-established and evolving area of cardiovascular diagnostic medical imaging. The prevalence of cardiac MRI, also termed CMR, is increasing in both conventional and specialty cardiovascular imaging. The use and indications for CMR grow as computing capabilities, protocol development, and research expand the potential for this imaging modality. In many areas, CMR is considered the reference standard owing to its high resolution, unlimited imaging planes, and ability to provide multiple types of information in a single study.

Despite these advantages of CMR, its use is not ubiquitous in cardiac diagnostics and treatment. Echocardiography, nuclear cardiology, and angiography remain

[a] Milton S. Hershey Medical Center, Penn State University, Mail Code H047, Room 1411, 500 University Drive, PO Box 850, Hershey, PA 17033-0850, USA; [b] Cardiovascular Magnetic Resonance Imaging, Temple University School of Medicine, PA, USA; [c] Allegheny General Hospital, Allegheny Health Network, Carnegie Mellon University, 320 East North Avenue, Pittsburgh, PA 15212, USA
* Corresponding author. Allegheny General Hospital, Allegheny Health Network, Carnegie Mellon University, 320 East North Avenue, Pittsburgh, PA 15212.
E-mail address: rbiedm@wpahs.org

Med Clin N Am 99 (2015) 849–861
http://dx.doi.org/10.1016/j.mcna.2015.02.011
0025-7125/15/$ – see front matter © 2015 Elsevier Inc. All rights reserved.

more active areas of cardiac imaging in most institutions. Issues such as availability of hardware and appropriately trained staff, prolonged study times, higher costs, patient safety, and patient compliance limit the role of CMR. In some circumstances, alternative imaging modalities or testing can provide similar information in an easier way, at a lesser cost, or with less need for specially trained staff.

Understanding the advantages CMR offers over other modalities and how these can improve diagnostic yield and patient management is central to appropriate utilization. Appropriateness criteria for CMR were established in the United States by a writing group of clinical and technical experts representing multiple major cardiovascular societies and groups.[1] This article was published in 2006 and although the technology and techniques are evolving, it covers a majority of the indications still most likely to be encountered in current practice. Other countries and major societies have released appropriateness criteria or reviews of clinical indications for CMR.[2–4] Most are more recent than the US document, but the indications are not significantly different. This reflects that much research is focused on validation and improvements in current imaging indications. At the same time, other research continues to expand the potential for CMR by investigating and validating new techniques and is likely to impact future indications for this imaging modality.

This article focuses on the well-established uses and indications for CMR in existing practice. The key clinical scenarios in which CMR is encountered in patient care are outlined. Attention is given to areas in which CMR excels in diagnostic cardiology as well as those in which it may be considered if more common imaging studies provide inadequate or conflicting information. Finally, some key safety issues for CMR are highlighted.

IMAGE ACQUISITION

To fully appreciate the use and application of CMR, a brief review of MRI acquisition and cardiac specific techniques is helpful. Routine CMR is performed on 1.5 T MRI scanners, which must be equipped with cardiac-specific hardware and software. An MRI scanner typically has its own room, and separate control and power rooms are also required. This space is more extensive than the equipment required for other imaging modalities. The patient is placed inside the MRI scanner for image acquisition. Phased array coils for receiving electromagnetic signal from the patient and electrocardiogram leads for monitoring the heart rate are placed on the patient.

In most MRIs, the magnetic field and associated gradients are created by superconducting, liquid helium–cooled electromagnets. In simplistic terms, the powerful magnetic fields from an MRI scanner affect the abundant hydrogen nuclei in the body, which act like miniature magnets. Gradients created by additional coils in the scanner cause a spatially related difference in how these hydrogen nuclei are affected. Radiofrequency (RF) pulses, also generated by the MRI scanner, can then be used to manipulate the hydrogen nuclei in select planes of any predetermined location and size. Owing to their magnetic properties, the hydrogen nuclei that are affected by the RF pulse will give off an electromagnetic signal that can be detected and, through a complex process known as Fourier transform, displayed as a 2-dimensional or 3-dimensional (3D) image. Each acquisition is based on the established position of the patient with respect to the magnetic field and gradients. Therefore, the patient cannot move the area of interest once the scan is started.

Most non-CMR consists of static images. To gain functional information throughout the cardiac cycle, dynamic time-resolved (cine) images are required. Real-time CMR, which would acquire an entire dynamic picture of the heart in a single heartbeat, is possible, but at the expense of reduced resolution. This is owing to limitations in how fast the magnetic gradients and RF pulses can be manipulated. Timing the CMR sequences to the electrocardiogram signal allows acquisition over multiple cardiac cycles, thereby improving resolution. To further improve quality of cine images, the patient is frequently instructed to hold their breath or perform controlled breathing. Free breathing images and respiratory gating are possible, but can prolong dramatically acquisition time and potentially affect resolution.

It is owing to these properties of MRI acquisition that the average study lasts longer than other imaging modalities, requires the patient to be still and compliant in an enclosed space, and is affected by irregular cardiac rhythms or limited respiratory reserve. These factors must be considered in the referral, planning, and preparation for a CMR.

IMAGING APPLICATIONS AND TECHNIQUES

The imaging applications and techniques available for CMR are abundant. In this section, the key clinical data available from a CMR study and the associated CMR acquisition techniques applied to obtain this information are reviewed. **Box 1** outlines these data and the associated CMR techniques, but is not all inclusive.

As outlined in **Box 1** and throughout the rest of this section, the potential for valuable information from CMR is immense. However, performing all possible CMR imaging on a single patient would result in a prohibitively long scan time. Depending on the known or suspected clinical condition, the images and techniques used in a CMR examination vary greatly. The composition of imaging techniques used in an individual scan is referred to as the acquisition protocol.

There is no single CMR acquisition protocol that is suitable for all clinical circumstances. The technologist and physician performing the CMR select the most appropriate imaging sequences to provide accurate and clinically useful information. The ordering physician must only supply the diagnosis or clinical question. Many centers have preset protocols for common scenarios that can be adjusted by the technologist and physician as needed. Not all hospitals and imaging centers are capable of performing all techniques based on hardware, software, and personnel available.

The most common imaging technique in CMR is cine imaging. All CMR acquisition protocols incorporate some component of cine imaging to provide moving images of the heart and surrounding structures. Ventricular function can be assessed by orienting views similar to those seen in echocardiography (**Fig. 1**A). In addition to traditional echo-centric views, CMR images can be obtained in any orientation. This flexibility allows assessment of the heart in views that are not possible by echocardiography owing to limitations of available acoustic windows (see **Fig. 1**B). These images permit assessment of regional wall motion, wall thickness, and abnormalities of the endocardium or other intracardiac structures. A stack of cine images that traverse the ventricular chambers can be used to quantify volumes, mass, and function without the need for geometric assumptions. To accomplish this, the endocardium and epicardium are traced in end diastole and end systole (see **Fig. 1**C). This is done frequently by hand, but semiautomated or completely automated programs are becoming more common.[5] In select cases, atrial volume and function can also be assessed. In addition to volumetric and functional analysis of the cardiac chambers, cine imaging can also be useful in assessing valve morphology and function, abnormal congenital anatomy or surgical repairs, the pericardium, vascular structures, and intracardiac or extracardiac masses. Myocardial tagging uses saturation bands across moving images to differentiate the relationship between structures, such as the pericardium or masses.

Box 1
CMR applications and techniques

Cardiac Volume, Mass, and Function

- 2D cine imaging
  - Traditional cardiac imaging planes to focus on:
    - Left ventricle
    - Right ventricle
    - Atria
    - Valves
  - Select orientations (limitless)
- Myocardial tagging

Cardiac structure and anatomy

- 2D static imaging
  - Axial, coronal, sagittal slices
  - Select orientations (limitless)

Blood flow quantification

- Velocity encoded imaging
  - Aorta
  - Pulmonary artery
  - Select orientations (limitless)

Tissue Characterization

- Late gadolinium enhancement
  - Fibrosis, scar, injury
- T1 weighting
  - Fatty deposition
- T2 weighting
  - Edema/inflammation
- T2* (T2-star)
  - Iron deposition
- Fat saturation

Angiography

- 3D imaging with focus on:
  - Aorta
  - Pulmonary artery
  - Pulmonary veins

Perfusion/stress imaging

- Resting perfusion
- Dobutamine stress function imaging
- Adenosine stress perfusion imaging

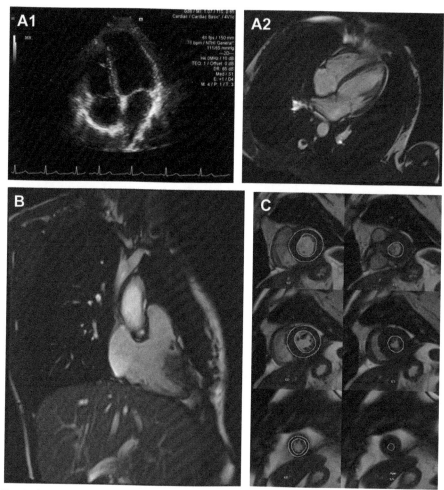

Fig. 1. (*A1, A2*) Compares transthoracic echocardiography (ECHO) and cardiac MR (CMR) 4-chamber views. (*B*) Right ventricular long axis view in CMR, not available by ECHO. (*C*) Select views from a staked short axis acquisition in diastole and systole with endocardial and epicardial tracing.

CMR is also capable of generating static images. These can be obtained more quickly than their cine counterparts, but are still gated so acquisition can occur at end diastole to reduce motion artifact. At a minimum, static images are obtained in axial, coronal, and sagittal planes in all patients to locate the body in relation to the scanner and serve as the reference for orientation of subsequent imaging planes. Like cine acquisitions, static imaging can also be obtained in any orientation and size.

Tissue characterization is the primary function of CMR that sets it apart from all other imaging modalities. Addition of contrast material as well as manipulation of the gradients, RF pulses, and the timing of signal acquisition can all be used to emphasize certain tissue characteristics in both cine and static imaging (**Fig. 2**). These various techniques can be used to establish the presence and potentially quantify the extent of tissue abnormalities in or around the cardiac muscle. These abnormalities can include myocardial fibrosis (see **Fig. 2**), edema, fatty infiltration, iron

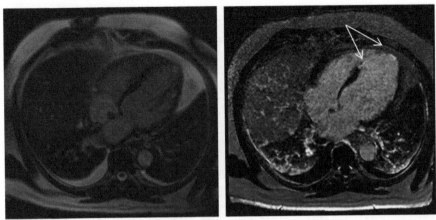

Fig. 2. Still frame from a 4-chamber cine acquisition on the left. Late gadolinium enhancement on a 4-chamber static acquisition from the same patient on the right. The bright signal in the ventricular wall from mid septum to apex (*arrows*) represent near-complete transmural fibrosis (*scar*) from a myocardial infarction.

deposition, thrombus, and tumor identification. Tissue characterization assists in the diagnosis or assessment of many cardiovascular conditions. Several of these uses are highlighted in the next section.

MR angiography to define and measure vascular anatomy is performed with 3D acquisition techniques and the use of a gadolinium intravenous contrast agent (**Fig. 3**). Noncontrast MR angiography is also possible. Blood flow through vessels

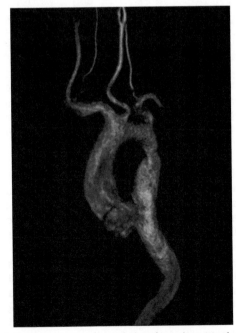

Fig. 3. Three-dimensional MR angiogram of the thoracic aorta in a patient with prior coarctation repair.

or valves can be quantified using velocity encoding. This technique results in differentiation of velocity, direction, and volume of blood flow and is particularly useful in quantitating valvular stenosis, regurgitation, and intracardiac shunts.

By using cine imaging with contrast injection and/or pharmacologic agents, CMR can assess coronary artery perfusion. Injection of contrast agent with visualization of the myocardium during the first pass through the circulation allows for visualization of resting perfusion. The same injection and visualization during pharmacologically induced vasodilation can assess for regional variations in flow associated with occlusive coronary artery disease. Similarly, cine image can be performed during dobutamine infusion to assess for regional wall motion abnormalities with pharmacologic stress. Owing to the importance of patient position in the magnet for image acquisition, physical exercise is not generally used for CMR stress perfusion or stress function imaging.

CLINICAL USES AND INDICATIONS

These sections each provide a brief overview of the major clinical areas and some specific conditions in which CMR can be applied. Each section opens with a table (**Tables 1–3**) that outlines the clinical uses and associated imaging techniques. Key CMR findings are summarized. The information is not exhaustive, but is designed to give a high level overview of current CMR utilization.

Cardiomyopathy (Nonischemic)

One of the more common roles for CMR is the differentiation and evaluation of nonischemic cardiomyopathies. CMR may be used in the acute setting of a patient who presents with positive cardiac enzymes or in the chronic evaluation of a patient with a reduced ejection fraction when there is minimal or no occlusive coronary artery disease. General evaluation consists of quantifying ventricular size and function as outlined in the previous section. By combining additional tissue characterization imaging sequences with and without the use of contrast enhancement, CMR is capable of further differentiating various types of nonischemic cardiomyopathies.[6,7] In many institutions, CMR is the test of choice for exceeding the inaccuracies of myocardial biopsy. In addition to diagnostic value, in many patients CMR findings also carry prognostic significance.[7]

Table 1
Cardiac MR in cardiomyopathies (nonischemic)

Clinical Uses	Imaging Techniques

• Differentiating from ischemic heart disease
• Acute myocarditis
• Hypertrophic cardiomyopathy
• Ventricular noncompaction
• Arrhythmogenic cardiomyopathy
• Cardiac sarcoidosis
• Cardiac amyloidosis
• Myocardial siderosis
	• Used in all cases:
	  ○ Cardiac volume, mass, and function
	    ■ 2D cine imaging
	  ○ Cardiac structure and anatomy
	    ■ 2D Static Imaging
	• Used in most cases:
	  ○ Flow
	  ○ Tissue characterization
	    ■ Late gadolinium enhancement
	• Used in select cases:
	  ○ Tissue characterization
	    ■ T1, T2, T2*, fat saturation
	  ○ Myocardial tagging
	  ○ Resting perfusion

Table 2
Cardiac MR in ischemic heart disease

Clinical Uses	Imaging Techniques

• Differentiating from nonischemic heart disease
• Acute coronary syndrome
• Viability
• Scar
• Remodeling
• Stress testing
• Anomalous coronary arteries
	• Used in all cases:
	  ○ Cardiac structure and anatomy
	    ■ 2D static imaging
	  ○ Cardiac volume, mass, and function
	    ■ 2D cine imaging
	• Used in most cases:
	  ○ Flow
	  ○ Tissue characterization
	    ■ Late gadolinium enhancement
	• Used in select cases:
	  ○ Tissue characterization
	    ■ T2
	  ○ Resting perfusion
	  ○ Dobutamine stress function imaging
	  ○ Adenosine stress perfusion imaging

CMR can play a central role in the diagnosis or confirmation of suspected myocarditis.[8] However, because many cases of myocarditis have a benign course with largely supportive care, CMR is not required in everyone with a suspected case. Ongoing symptoms, evidence of myocardial injury, and a history consistent with an infectious or inflammatory etiology should be present to consider CMR.[8] No single finding confirms or excludes myocarditis with complete certainty. Typically a protocol that uses several tissue characterization techniques designed to assess for inflammation and/or irreversible injury is applied to rule out or establish the diagnosis of acute myocarditis.[9] In suspected myocarditis, normal findings on a CMR correlate with a good prognosis.[10]

In hypertrophic cardiomyopathy (HCM), CMR is used to quantify regional and global left ventricular (LV) mass. This may be most helpful in patients with ambiguous findings on echocardiography or suspected atypical HCM patterns.[11] Tissue characterization with late gadolinium enhancement displays fibrosis. In HCM, this is seen most often at the site of right ventricle (RV) insertion into the LV and within the most pronounced regions of hypertrophy. In addition to anatomic findings, the presence and extent of fibrosis may help in predicting HCM patients at greatest risk for sudden cardiac death.[12]

Table 3
Cardiac MR in intracardiac and extracardiac structures

Clinical Uses	Imaging Techniques

• Cardiac masses
  ○ Benign tumors
  ○ Malignant tumors
  ○ Thrombus
• Pericardial conditions
• Vascular structures
  ○ Aorta
  ○ Pulmonary artery
  ○ Pulmonary veins
	• Used in all cases:
	  ○ Cardiac structure and anatomy
	    ■ 2D static imaging
	  ○ Cardiac volume, mass, and function
	    ■ 2D cine imaging
	• Used in select cases:
	  ○ Tissue characterization
	    ■ T1, T2, late gadolinium enhancement
	  ○ Resting perfusion
	  ○ Myocardial tagging
	  ○ Flow
	  ○ Angiography

Ventricular noncompaction is defined by the abnormal ratio of a thin compacted layer of myocardium and a larger thick layer of noncompacted myocardium. MRI of the heart is used to further evaluate suspected cases. The ratio between compacted and noncompacted myocardium on CMR has been shown to distinguish pathologic LV noncompaction.[13]

Volumetric and functional assessment of the RV takes precedence in the assessment of arrhythmogenic right ventricular cardiomyopathy. RV-focused cine images are easier to obtain than with echocardiogram. Tissue characterization may play an important role by identifying fatty infiltration and fibrosis in the RV.[14]

In addition to the nonischemic cardiomyopathies listed, certain patterns of late gadolinium enhancement and tissue characterization can assist in the differentiation of other cardiomyopathies. Sarcoidosis, amyloidosis, and iron overload all have suggestive patterns on CMR examination.[7]

Ischemic Heart Disease

As with nonischemic cardiomyopathies, cardiac volume and function are integral to the assessment of ischemic heart disease. CMR has been considered the reference standard for volumetric and functional quantification for more than 20 years. This information may be feasible by more prevalent imaging modalities, particularly echocardiography, but CMR is appropriate to consider when other data are insufficient, unavailable, or discrepant.[1]

The assessment of myocardial scar and fibrosis is a more common reason for CMR in ischemic heart disease. Tissue characterization with late gadolinium enhancement techniques can detect changes in both acute and chronic myocardial infarction. The high resolution capabilities of CMR allow it to distinguish between subendocardial and transmural infarctions and detect infarction in the relatively thin RV walls. The extent of infarction as a percentage of the complete wall thickness in the LV correlates with myocardial viability and the likelihood of functional recovery after revascularization.[15]

In a properly equipped center, stress function and perfusion imaging can be done as a part of the CMR study to assess for coronary artery disease. Stress CMR has been shown to be equal or superior to dobutamine stress echocardiography and vasodilator stress in the detection of hemodynamically significant coronary artery disease.[6] It has also been demonstrated to have prognostic value.[16] A recent pivotal trial is emblematic of the capability of CMR in this area. When compared with nuclear radioisotope approaches in this large prospective study, CMR had greater sensitivity and better negative predictive value in predicting the presence of coronary artery disease as defined by subsequent angiography.[17] Other stress testing modalities are often more accessible, but this trial and others have led many centers to reconsider low-resolution imaging when highly resolved CMR is available.

Although CMR is not used commonly to directly assess coronary artery disease by imaging stenosis severity or composition, it is appropriate as a noninvasive method for detecting suspected anomalous coronary arteries in young patients without the need for ionizing radiation.[1]

Intracardiac and Extracardiac Structures

Suspected cardiac masses may be benign, malignant, or ultimately found to be artifact. Protocols for cardiac masses use multiple tissue characterization sequences, resting perfusion, and occasionally myocardial tagging. CMR excels in defining their location and extent. It many instances, it can suggest a most likely diagnosis.

CMR is able to assess accurately pericardial conditions that may be difficult to detect or quantify by other imaging modalities. Echocardiography can visualize and assess many pericardial conditions. CMR can provide incremental value over echocardiography for assessment of pericardial thickening, masses, and loculated or complex effusions because of its unlimited imaging planes and high resolution. CT is the first-line modality for assessing pericardial calcium, but CMR's ability to simultaneously assess functional data makes it more desirable than CT in most other pericardial conditions, especially for delineation of constrictive pericarditis and the need for percardiectomy.

Magnetic resonance angiography with 3D acquisitions allow for the reconstruction of and measurement of vascular structures. Similar techniques are used to recreate the left atrium in preparation for electrophysiology procedures such as pulmonary vein isolation.

Other Uses for Cardiac Magnetic Resonance

Valvular heart disease evaluation can be aided by CMR, particularly when echocardiography imaging is suboptimal. CMR offers visualization of the valve structure and function with cine imaging. Flow quantification can be helpful for quantifying regurgitant volumes and stenotic gradients. Both techniques are of value for assessing valvular lesions.[18] Ventricular volume and function by CMR, as highlighted throughout the preceding sections, may be useful to guide interventions.

CMR is uniquely well-suited for the evaluation of congenital heart disease patients. The capabilities of CMR to provide high-resolution imaging not limited by traditional echocardiographic imaging views, assess volume and function with high reproducibility, evaluate valvular disease, perform angiography, and characterize fibrosis and scarring all without ionizing radiation make it ideal in this population. Owing to the complex and diverse nature of most congenital heart disease, a more thorough review of CMR applications and techniques in this population is beyond the scope of this review.

SAFETY
Implanted Devices and Foreign Bodies

MRI scanning involves no ionizing radiation or biological effects on the body. It is noninvasive except for the possibility of a peripheral intravenous line for contrast administration. The major safety risk with any MRI study is related to the presence of implanted devices or foreign bodies in the patient that have ferromagnetic properties. Except in a few circumstances, guidelines for the MRI safety of devices and foreign bodies are not a simple set of broad "yes" and "no" categories. For this reason, even many medical professionals may not know specific safety information. This gap in knowledge can lead to requests for unsafe examinations or deferment of appropriate studies. Many of the limited cases of MRI-related injuries and deaths have resulted from failure to follow recognized safety guidelines.[19]

In general, nonferromagnetic materials can be safely scanned at any time. Weakly ferromagnetic materials should be considered on a case-by-case basis and require a careful risk benefit analysis and discussion with the patient. Strongly ferromagnetic materials are typically contraindicated in the MRI scanner. In select cases, patients with ferromagnetic cardiac devices (pacemakers, automatic internal cardiac defibrillators) may undergo MRI under proper supervision if the risk of not performing the study is felt to outweigh the risk of the examination.[20] It is beyond the scope of this review to cover specifically the safety of individual devices, but a general list of categories is found in **Table 4**. This list is predominantly derived from information contained in the following 2 sources:

Table 4
Common implanted devices and foreign bodies

Cardiac Devices	Noncardiac Devices/Foreign Bodies
Coronary artery stents: MRI safe	Peripheral vascular stents: most MRI safe; some MRI conditional
Sternal wires: MRI safe	
Prosthetic cardiac valves and annuloplasty rings: most MRI safe; some MRI conditional	Inferior vena cava filters: most MRI safe; some MRI conditional
Cardiac closure and occlusion devices: most MRI safe; several MRI conditional	Embolization coils: most MRI safe; some MRI conditional
Loop Recorder: MRL conditional (download all stored data before MRI)	Aneurysm clips: vary by type
Pacemarker/automatic internal cardiac defibrillator: generally MRI unsafe[a]	Aortic stent grafts: most MRI safe; some MRI conditional; some MRI unsafe
Temporary pacing devices: MRI unsafe	Orthopedic implants: many are MRI safe or MRI contitional; some MRI unsafe
Indwelling hemodynamic monitors (Swann Ganz catheters): MRI unsafe	Transdermal patches: MRI unsafe if they contain metals in their backing
Hemodynamic support devices: MRI unsafe (limited data)	Ocular metal shavings: MRI unsafe

[a] Some recent devices approved for MRI use.

- Safety of Magnetic Resonance Imaging in Patients with Cardiovascular Devices. A statement paper published by the AHA in 2007[19] and
- http://www.mrisafety.com/.[21]

All patients undergoing an MRI require a thorough safety screen, which should be performed by the staff at the MRI facility before an examination is performed. This safety screen typically involves a questionnaire, background check of any implanted devices or foreign materials, and a metal detector screening before entering the magnet room.

Contrast Agents

Gadolinium, the contrast agent delivered for angiography and tissue enhancement in CMR, is not nephrotoxic, but should be administered with caution in patients with renal failure owing to the potential for the rare but serious side effect of nephrogenic systemic fibrosis. A preprocedure creatinine level and creatinine clearance estimate is performed before contrast is administered.

Pregnancy

The risk of an MRI for a developing fetus is unknown, but is generally felt to be safe. It does not deliver any ionizing radiation to the unborn child. Gadolinium does cross the placenta and is generally not recommended in pregnancy.

SUMMARY

CMR is a highly capable and diverse cardiovascular imaging tool. It serves as the reference standard in many areas, but is not always standard of care owing to limitations imposed by availability, cost effectiveness, and safety. Appropriateness criteria have been defined, but are likely to evolve with advances in techniques and ongoing validation research. Understanding the basics of CMR acquisition techniques and the broad categories of appropriate applications will assist with selecting the best clinical scenarios to consider CMR.

REFERENCES

1. Hendel RC, Patel MR, Kramer CM, et al. ACCF/ACR/SCCT/SCMR/ASNC/NASCI/SCAI/SIR 2006 appropriateness criteria for cardiac computed tomography and cardiac magnetic resonance imaging: a report of the American College of Cardiology Foundation Quality Strategic Directions Committee Appropriateness Criteria Working Group, American College of Radiology, Society of Cardiovascular Computed Tomography, Society for Cardiovascular Magnetic Resonance, American Society of Nuclear Cardiology, North American Society for Cardiac Imaging, Society for Cardiovascular Angiography and Interventions, and Society of Interventional Radiology. J Am Coll Cardiol 2006;48:1475–97.
2. Pennell DJ, Sechtem UP, Higgins CB, et al. Clinical indications for cardiovascular magnetic resonance (CMR): consensus panel report. Eur Heart J 2004;25:1940–65.
3. Di Cesare E, Cademartiri F, Carbone I, et al. Clinical indications for the use of cardiac MRI. By the SIRM Study Group on Cardiac Imaging. Radiol Med 2013;118:752–98 [in Italian].
4. Hergan K, Globits S, Schuchlenz H, et al. Clinical relevance and indications for cardiac magnetic resonance imaging 2013: an interdisciplinary expert statement. Rofo 2013;185:209–18 [in German].
5. Attili AK, Schuster A, Nagel E, et al. Quantification in cardiac MRI: advances in image acquisition and processing. Int J Cardiovasc Imaging 2010;26(Suppl 1):27–40.
6. Beach S, Syed MA. Current and upcoming roles of CT and MRI in clinical cardiac imagery. Curr Cardiol Rep 2007;9:420–7.
7. Steel KE, Kwong RY. Application of cardiac magnetic resonance imaging in cardiomyopathy. Curr Heart Fail Rep 2008;5:128–35.
8. Friedrich MG, Sechtem U, Schulz-Menger J, et al. Cardiovascular magnetic resonance in myocarditis: a JACC white paper. J Am Coll Cardiol 2009;53:1475–87.
9. Laissy JP, Messin B, Varenne O, et al. MRI of acute myocarditis: a comprehensive approach based on various imaging sequences. Chest 2002;122:1638–48.
10. Schumm J, Greulich S, Wagner A, et al. Cardiovascular magnetic resonance risk stratification in patients with clinically suspected myocarditis. J Cardiovasc Magn Reson 2014;16:14.
11. To AC, Dhillon A, Desai MY. Cardiac magnetic resonance in hypertrophic cardiomyopathy. JACC Cardiovasc Imaging 2011;4:1123–37.
12. Kwon DH, Desai MY. Cardiac magnetic resonance in hypertrophic cardiomyopathy: current state of the art. Expert Rev Cardiovasc Ther 2010;8:103–11.
13. Petersen SE, Selvanayagam JB, Wiesmann F, et al. Left ventricular noncompaction: insights from cardiovascular magnetic resonance imaging. J Am Coll Cardiol 2005;46:101–5.
14. Tandri H, Macedo R, Calkins H, et al. Role of magnetic resonance imaging in arrhythmogenic right ventricular dysplasia: insights from the North American arrhythmogenic right ventricular dysplasia (ARVD/C) study. Am Heart J 2008;155:147–53 [Erratum appears in Am Heart J 2008;155(2):289].
15. Selvanayagam JB, Kardos A, Francis JM, et al. Value of delayed-enhancement cardiovascular magnetic resonance imaging in predicting myocardial viability after surgical revascularization. Circulation 2004;110:1535–41.
16. Jahnke C, Nagel E, Gebker R, et al. Prognostic value of cardiac magnetic resonance stress tests: adenosine stress perfusion and dobutamine stress wall motion imaging. Circulation 2007;115:1769–76.

17. Greenwood JP, Maredia N, Younger JF, et al. Cardiovascular magnetic resonance and single-photon emission computed tomography for diagnosis of coronary heart disease (CE-MARC): a prospective trial. Lancet 2012;379:453–60.
18. Reddy ST, Shah M, Doyle M, et al. Evaluation of cardiac valvular regurgitant lesions by cardiac MRI sequences: comparison of a four-valve semi-quantitative versus quantitative approach. J Heart Valve Dis 2013;22:491–9.
19. Levine GN, Gomes AS, Arai AE, et al. Safety of magnetic resonance imaging in patients with cardiovascular devices: an American Heart Association Scientific Statement From the Committee on Diagnostic and Interventional Cardiac Catheterization, Council on Clinical Cardiology, and the Council on Cardiovascular Radiology and Intervention: Endorsed by the American College of Cardiology Foundation, the North American Society for Cardiac Imaging, and the Society for Cardiovascular Magnetic Resonance. Circulation 2007;116:2878–91.
20. Biederman RW, Doyle M, Yamrozik J. The cardiovascular MRI tutorial: lectures and learning. Philadelphia: Lippincott Williams & Wilkins; 2008.
21. MRI Safety Website. Available at: http://www.mrisafety.com/. Accessed September 18, 2014.

Current Management of Heart Failure

When to Refer to Heart Failure Specialist and When Hospice is the Best Option

Behnam Bozorgnia, MD[a], Paul J. Mather, MD[b],*

KEYWORDS

- Acute and chronic management • Heart failure • Hospital care • Hospice care

KEY POINTS

- Heart failure is a common symptom caused by variety of pathologies.
- Management of heart failure should be tailored to the specific pathology.
- Level of care for heart failure should be escalated as the disease progresses to more advanced stages.

Heart failure (HF) is a common syndrome caused by different abnormalities of the cardiovascular system that result in impairment of the ventricles in filling or ejecting blood. HF is one of the most common causes of hospitalization in the United States with a very high cost to the health care system. In the United States there are 880,000 new HF diagnoses per year and 5 million cases currently identified.[1–3] This article focuses on the etiology of left ventricle dysfunction, HF presentation, and the acute and chronic management of HF.

ETIOLOGY OF HEART FAILURE

There is a broad spectrum of disorders that cause left ventricular dysfunction. The etiologic spectrum of systolic and diastolic dysfunction ranges from coronary artery disease, hypertension, and valvular heart disease, to more rare causes such as infiltrative disorders and parasitic infections. **Box 1** lists the most common causes of HF encountered by clinicians.

[a] Advanced Heart Failure and Mechanical Circulatory Support, Einstein Medical Center, Moss Building, 3rd Floor, 5501 Old York Road, Philadelphia, PA 19141, USA; [b] Advanced Heart Failure and Cardiac Transplant Center, The Jefferson Heart Institute, Jefferson Medical College of Thomas Jefferson University, 925 Chestnut Street, Suite 323A, Philadelphia, PA 19107, USA
* Corresponding author.
E-mail address: Paul.Mather@jefferson.edu

Med Clin N Am 99 (2015) 863–876
http://dx.doi.org/10.1016/j.mcna.2015.02.012
0025-7125/15/$ – see front matter © 2015 Elsevier Inc. All rights reserved.

Box 1
Etiology of heart failure

There is no agreed or satisfactory classification for the causes of heart failure, with much overlap between potential categories

Myocardial disease

1. Coronary artery disease

2. Hypertension[a]

3. Cardiomyopathy[b]

   a. Familial

      i. Hypertrophic

      ii. Dilated

      iii. Arrhythmogenic right ventricular cardiomyopathy

      iv. Restrictive

      v. Left ventricular noncompaction

   b. Acquired

      i. Myocarditis (inflammatory cardiomyopathy)

         Infective

- Bacterial
- Spirochetal
- Fungal
- Protozoal
- Parasitic
- Rickettsial
- Viral

         Immune mediated

- Tetanus toxoid, vaccines, serum sickness
- Drugs
- Lymphocytic/giant cell myocarditis
- Sarcoidosis
- Autoimmune
- Eosinophilic (Churg-Strauss)

         Toxic

- Drugs (eg, chemotherapy, cocaine)
- Alcohol
- Heavy metals (copper, iron, lead)

      ii. Endocrine/nutritional

- Pheochromocytoma
- Vitamin deficiency (eg, thiamine)
- Selenium deficiency
- Hypophosphatemia
- Hypocalcemia

    iii. Pregnancy

    iv. Infiltration

      • Amyloidosis

      • Malignancy

Valvular heart disease

  Mitral

  Aortic

  Tricuspid

  Pulmonary

Pericardial disease

  Constrictive pericarditis

  Pericardial effusion

Endocardial disease

• Endomyocardial diseases with hypereosinophilia (hypereosinophilic syndromes [HES])

• Endomyocardial disease without hypereosinophilia (eg, endomyocardial fibrosis [EMF])

• Endocardial fibroelastosis

Congenital heart disease

  Arrhythmia

    Tachyarrhythmia

      Atrial

      Ventricular

    Bradyarrhythmia

      Sinus node dysfunction

Conduction disorders

• Atrioventricular block

High-output states

• Anemia

• Sepsis

• Thyrotoxicosis

• Paget disease

• Arteriovenous fistula

Volume overload

• Renal failure

• Iatrogenic (eg, postoperative fluid infusion)

  [a] Both peripheral arterial and myocardial factors contribute to the development of heart failure.

  [b] Other inherited diseases may have cardiac effects, eg, Fabry disease.

  Adapted from McMurray JJ, Adamopoulos S, Anker SD, et al. ESC Guidelines for the diagnosis and treatment of acute and chronic heart failure 2012. The Task Force for the Diagnosis and Treatment of Acute and Chronic Heart Failure 2012 of the European Society of Cardiology. Developed in collaboration with the Heart Failure Association (HFA) of the ESC. Eur Heart J 2012;33(14):1787–847.

ACUTE HEART FAILURE

Common presenting symptoms of HF can include mild shortness of breath, peripheral edema and fatigue, and more severe symptoms such as hypotension, syncope, shock, and respiratory failure. A thorough history and physical examination is critical in the diagnosis and treatment of patients with HF. The presence of risk factors for developing HF such as coronary artery disease, hypertension, and diabetes, and the presence of substance abuse or recent viral syndrome, can provide clues regarding causation. Exposure to chemotherapeutic agents, endocrine abnormalities, recent pregnancy, and a family history of HF or transplantation are all factors that should be addressed during the initial interview of the patient with HF. A comprehensive history will narrow down the extensive list of causes and allows the clinician to provide a more focused and tailored therapy.

Physical Examination

Vital signs

Evaluation of the HF patient starts with the vital signs. An elevated temperature can be present in myocarditis, or acute valvular lesions in infective endocarditis. Heart rate and regularity is also an imperative parameter in evaluating a patient with HF. Presence of tachycardia is an important and often ominous finding in acutely decompensated HF. Blood pressure can vary significantly depending on the stage and severity of the disease. HF patients can present to emergency room with very high systolic and diastolic pressures and acute pulmonary edema. A narrow pulse pressure (<25%) is a sign of low cardiac output and a severely decompensated HF patient.

The patient's state of mind and clarity can be determined during the interview. Low cardiac output can manifest itself as a confused patient who is difficult to arouse. Evaluation of the jugular venous pressure (JVP) is probably the most important and challenging part of the examination. JVP will determine the volume status of the patient, which will guide the HF therapy. JVP can also differentiate intravascular volume overload from extravascular edema present in other conditions. Presence of rales in an acute setting is common, although the absence of rales does not rule out HF, especially in a patient with chronic HF. The cardiac examination includes the regularity of the rhythm, and the presence of murmurs and gallops. A displaced point of maximal impulse indicates an enlarged heart. The abdominal examination includes the size of the liver and the presence of edema. Ascites and sacral, scrotal, or lower extremity edema can be present in a volume-overloaded patient with manifestations of right-sided HF. Cool extremities and low pulse volume can be another sign of the hypoperfused patient with low cardiac output. Palpation of the peripheral pulses can also be helpful in assessing cardiac performance and stroke volume. A full and round pulse, as compared with a short and pointed pulse, can be the difference between a compensated HF patient and a sign of low cardiac output, respectively.

Diagnostic Tests

Chest radiograph

Chest radiograph findings can be specific but not sensitive for diagnosing HF. Classically the presence of Kerley B lines, peribronchial cuffing, pleural effusions, and cephalization of the pulmonary vasculature can be present in HF patients.

Electrocardiogram

The electrocardiogram (ECG) determines the presence of any arrhythmias that are common in HF patients. Presence of Q waves, or ischemic changes such as ST elevation or depressions, versus left ventricular hypertrophy or low voltage may guide the clinician toward the correct etiology.

Laboratory data
Patients with acute HF can present with low sodium levels. Blood urea nitrogen (BUN)/creatinine can also be abnormal depending of the degree of decompensation and hypoperfusion. B-Type natriuretic peptide (BNP) or N-terminal pro-B-type natriuretic peptide (NT-proBNP) measurements are useful in an acutely decompensated patient.[4,5] Although the absolute value of each laboratory value can be variable, both BNP and NT-proBNP can be useful in distinguishing HF from other common conditions when the clinical picture is not clear (Class I indication). Of note, BNP levels can be falsely low in morbidly obese patients.

Other laboratory values to consider are:

- Troponin
- Thyroid-stimulating hormone
- Iron studies
- HIV
- Liver function test

Troponin levels can be elevated in both ischemic and nonischemic HF patients. Persistent elevation of troponin levels has a poor prognostic value in HF patients.[6] Liver function can also be a marker of the level of congestion and chronicity of HF. In appropriate patients, HIV and iron level are helpful in further narrowing down the possible causes of HF.

Acute Heart Failure Therapy

Once the underlying cause of HF is identified, the therapy can be tailored to the individual patient. When evaluating a patient with acute HF, it is important to assess the level of congestion (ie, wet versus dry) and the level of perfusion (ie, warm versus cold). The levels of congestion and perfusion of the HF patient will guide the initial therapy. **Fig. 1** provides a quick assessment of the hemodynamic profile of the HF patient.

Diuretics
Diuretic therapy is initiated in the acute setting to alleviate symptoms. Parenteral diuretic therapy should be initiated in an acute setting in a congested patient with adequate perfusion. The diuretic dose should be adjusted frequently until adequate response is obtained. The most commonly used loop diuretic is furosemide. Other diuretics such as bumetanide or torsemide are also used for their increased bioavailability in the oral form.

The diuretic effect of loop diuretics can be enhanced by addition of thiazide diuretics such as metolazone or spironolactone in a diuretic-resistant patient.[7] Renal function and electrolytes need to be monitored closely during aggressive parenteral diuresis.

When comparing intravenous bolus with continuous infusion of loop diuretics, the data have not shown a significant difference between the 2 strategies.[8] The clinician, however, can choose either method if the patient is refractory to the initial therapy.

Parenteral vasodilators
Parenteral vasodilators are used as adjuvant therapy to diuretics to relieve congestion and dyspnea in acute HF patients without hypotension. This class of medications increases systemic perfusion, including the renal system, and therefore enhances the diuretic effect of loop diuretics.

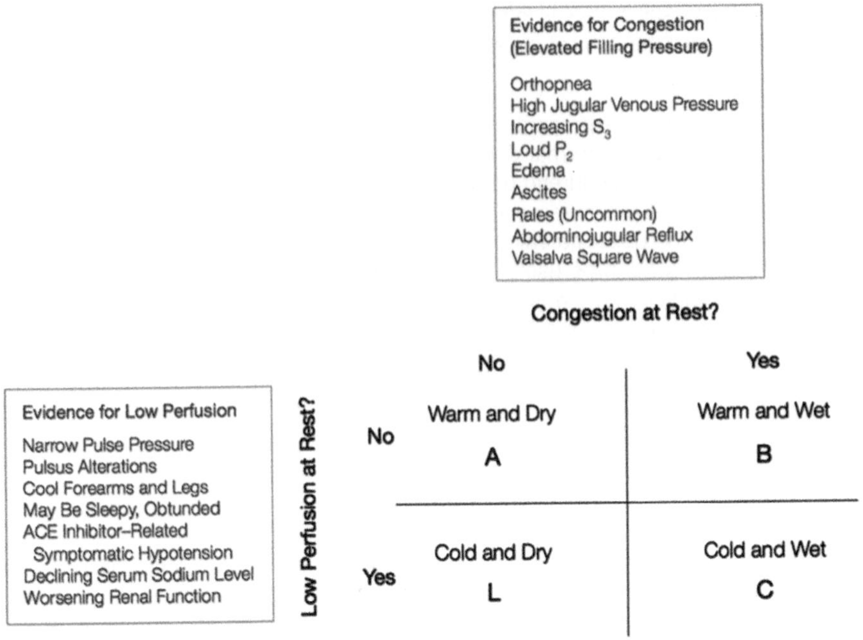

Evidence for Congestion (Elevated Filling Pressure)
Orthopnea High Jugular Venous Pressure Increasing S_3 Loud P_2 Edema Ascites Rales (Uncommon) Abdominojugular Reflux Valsalva Square Wave

Congestion at Rest?

		No	Yes
		Warm and Dry	Warm and Wet
Low Perfusion at Rest?	No	A	B
	Yes	Cold and Dry L	Cold and Wet C

Evidence for Low Perfusion

Narrow Pulse Pressure
Pulsus Alterations
Cool Forearms and Legs
May Be Sleepy, Obtunded
ACE Inhibitor–Related
  Symptomatic Hypotension
Declining Serum Sodium Level
Worsening Renal Function

Fig. 1. A quick assessment of the hemodynamic profile is critical before initiation of therapy because the spectrum of therapy can be variable and wide. The patient with profile A (warm and dry) can be managed as an outpatient, whereas patients with profile C (cold/wet) will need inotrope or mechanical circulatory support. ACE, angiotensin-converting enzyme. (*Courtesy of* A. Nohria, MD, E. Lewis, MD, and LW Stevenson, MD, Boston MA; with permission.)

Intravenous nitroglycerin can relieve congestion primarily through venodilation. This agent is mainly used in hypertensive patients with pulmonary edema, and can also relieve symptoms of angina in patients with significant coronary disease. This agent is usually effective in up to 24 hours. Patients can develop tachyphylaxis or resistance to nitroglycerin during this time.[9]

Sodium nitroprusside is another potent vasodilator used to treat acute HF. This medication relieves congestion by dilating the venous and arterial beds and reducing the systemic vascular resistance. Arterial line hemodynamic monitoring is usually needed during therapy, as nitroprusside can cause precipitous hypotension. Rare thiocyanate toxicity can occur with prolonged use, particularly in patients with renal impairment.[10]

Nesiritide can also be used to relieve symptoms of dyspnea and enhance diuresis in acute HF. As with the vasodilators already mentioned, hypotension is a side effect during therapy. BNP levels are not reliable during administration of nesiritide. It is also noteworthy that the aforesaid vasodilators have not shown any mortality benefit for HF patients and are only used in the acute setting for symptomatic relief.[11]

β-Blockers

β-Blockers (BBs) represent an important class of drugs used in the treatment of HF.[12] In an acute presentation of HF, however, their use requires some clinical judgment and finesse. BBs can be initiated at a low dose, or continued if the patient is already on BB therapy as an outpatient, in a well-perfused patient. Titration of this class of drugs, however, should be avoided during the acute phase of HF. The dose of BB should be reduced or stopped in more severe presentations of HF. It is imperative, however, that the patient be initiated on BB therapy before discharge to ensure its use as transitions of care occur.

Sinus tachycardia is often present in acute HF presentation. One should refrain from titrating the BB dose to suppress sinus tachycardia in HF. In acutely decompensated HF, sinus tachycardia is an appropriate and crucial physiologic response to a state of low cardiac output. Sinus tachycardia is usually resolved as the hemodynamic profile of the HF patient improves.

The literature on HF and BBs is extensive, although results with certain BB medications are mixed. For this reason, current recommendations encourage clinicians to use 1 of the 3 BBs that have showed benefit in clinical trials: bisoprolol, metoprolol succinate, or carvedilol. **Table 1** lists the target doses of the BBs in the treatment of HF.[12–15]

Angiotensin-converting enzyme inhibitors

Angiotensin-converting enzyme (ACE) inhibitors are the cornerstone of HF therapy.[16,17] The vasodilation effects of ACE inhibitors are key in improving hemodynamics of HF in both acute and chronic states. Unlike BBs, ACE inhibitors do exhibit a class effect. In acute HF patients without shock or significant renal dysfunction, ACE inhibitors should be initiated at low dose and titrated to the maximum tolerated dose. Short-acting ACE inhibitors such as captopril can be initiated in the acute setting if there is concern about hypotensive response. If tolerated, the short-acting captopril should be switched to a comparable dose of a long-acting ACE inhibitor such as lisinopril or enalapril. **Table 1** lists the target doses of ACE inhibitors in the treatment of HF.

Angiotensin-receptor blockers

Angiotensin-receptor blockers (ARBs) are also vasodilators that can be used instead of ACE inhibitors in patients with acute HF.[18–20] ARBs are used when patients exhibit ACE-inhibitor intolerance such as cough. **Table 1** Lists the target doses of the ARBs in the treatment of HF.

Aldosterone antagonists

Utility of aldosterone antagonists such as spironolactone or eplerenone are limited in an acute HF setting, and are further discussed in the section on chronic HF. Aldosterone antagonists facilitate the diuretic effect of loop diuretics in a congested HF patient.[21,22]

Hydralazine/nitrates

In HF patients with significant renal dysfunction or uncontrolled hypertension despite a maximum dose of ACE and BBs, afterload reducers such as a combination of hydralazine and nitrates can be used. Although the benefit of hydralazine/nitrates combination has been shown mostly in the African American population, this combination should be considered in non–African Americans when ACE inhibitors or ARBs are not tolerated, or resistant hypertension is present.[23]

Digoxin

Perhaps one of the oldest medications available, digoxin still has a role in the treatment of HF. Digoxin is also the only safe and effective oral inotropic agent identified thus far. Although this medication does not affect mortality, it has been shown to reduce hospitalization in HF patients.[24] The ideal use for digoxin is in patients with HF with reduced ejection fraction (HFrEF) with concomitant atrial fibrillation. Digoxin has a narrow therapeutic index, and its serum levels should be kept at 0.5 to 0.9 ng/mL. The dose of this medication should be reduced in renally impaired patients.

Table 1
Drugs commonly used in stage C heart failure with reduced ejection fraction

Drug	Initial Daily Dose(s)	Maximum Dose(s)	Mean Doses Achieved in Clinical Trials
ACE Inhibitors			
Captopril	6.25 mg 3 times	50 mg 3 times	122.7 mg/d (422)
Enalapril	2.5 mg twice	10–20 mg twice	16.6 mg/d (413)
Fosinopril	5–10 mg once	40 mg once	N/A
Lisinopril	2.5–5 mg once	20–40 mg once	32.5–35.0 mg/d (445)
Perindopril	2 mg once	8–16 mg once	N/A
Quinapril	5 mg twice	20 mg twice	N/A
Ramipril	1.25–2.5 mg once	10 mg once	N/A
Trandolapril	1 mg once	4 mg once	N/A
ARBs			
Candesartan	4–8 mg once	32 mg once	24 mg/d (420)
Losartan	25–50 mg once	50–150 mg once	129 mg/d (421)
Valsartan	20–40 mg twice	160 mg twice	254 mg/d (108)
Aldosterone Antagonists			
Spironolactone	12.5–25.0 mg once	25 mg once or twice	26 mg/d (425)
Eplerenone	25 mg once	50 mg once	42.6 mg/d (446)
β-Blockers			
Bisoprolol	1.25 mg once	10 mg once	8.6 mg/d (117)
Carvedilol	3.125 mg twice	50 mg twice	37 mg/d (447)
Carvedilol CR	10 mg once	80 mg once	N/A
Metoprolol succinate extended release (metoprolol CR/XL)	12.5–25 mg once	200 mg once	159 mg/d (448)
Hydralazine and Isosorbide Dinitrate			
Fixed-dose combination (424)	37.5 mg hydralazine/ 20 mg isosorbide dinitrate 3 times daily	75 mg hydralazine/ 40 mg isosorbide dinitrate 3 times daily	~175 mg hydralazine/ 90 mg isosorbide dinitrate daily
Hydralazine and isosorbide dinitrate (449)	Hydralazine: 25–50 mg, 3 or 4 times daily and isosorbide dinitrate: 20–30 mg 3 or 4 times daily	Hydralazine: 300 mg daily in divided doses and isosorbide dinitrate 120 mg daily in divided doses	N/A

Abbreviations: ACE, angiotensin-converting enzyme; ARB, angiotensin-receptor blocker; CR, controlled release; CR/XL, controlled release/extended release; N/A, not applicable.
Adapted from Yancy CW, Jessup M, Bozkurt B, et al. ACCF/AHA Guideline for the Management of Heart Failure: a report of the American College of Cardiology Foundation/American Heart Association Task Force on Practice Guidelines. Circulation 2013;128:1810–52; with permission.

Inotropes

Inotropic therapy is reserved for severely decompensated HF patients with signs of shock or hypoperfusion organ injury. Low cardiac output or shock, such as low pulse pressure, tachycardia, hypotension, and cool extremities, can be obvious. In some cases, however, signs of low cardiac output can be subtle, such as worsening of renal function with loop diuretics in a congested patient, changes in mental status, or abnormal liver function tests. Invasive hemodynamic monitoring is usually required to assess and manage patients with low cardiac output or shock. This section discusses the commonly used inotropic agents.

Milrinone Phosphodiesterase (PD) inhibitors block the degradation of cyclic adenosine monophosphate, leading to an increase in calcium influx into the myocardium and enhancement of contractility. PD inhibitors also have a vasodilatory effect on the pulmonary and peripheral circulation. Intravenous milrinone can be considered in HF patients with low cardiac output. This medication should be initiated at low dose and titrated to achieve acceptable hemodynamics. Because members of this class of drugs are also potent vasodilators, their use should be avoided in severely hypotensive patients. Concomitant use of low-dose BBs is possible with this class of medications because they increase contractility independent of the β-adrenergic pathway.[25]

Dobutamine β-Adrenergic receptor agonists can also provide enhanced contractility and hemodynamic support in severely decompensated HF patients with low cardiac output. Compared with PD inhibitors, dobutamine has a less vasodilatory effect on the periphery and is the preferred agent in hypotensive patients. Concomitant use of BBs, specially the nonselective class, should be avoided, as they counteract utilization of the same receptor.

In general, the use of intravenous inotropes is a temporary measure to provide hemodynamic support as a bridge to recovery or advanced therapies (transplant or left ventricular assist device [LVAD]). Long-term use of inotropes should be avoided except as palliative therapy in stage D HF patients, once all available therapies have been exhausted.[26,27]

Use of agents with both inotropic and vasopressor properties, such as norepinephrine, should only be used in profoundly hypotensive patients with hemodynamic collapse or sepsis. Pure vasopressors such as phenylephrine should generally be avoided in HF patients.

Mechanical circulatory support

In critically ill HF patients with severe hemodynamic compromise who are not responsive to medical therapy, mechanical circulatory support (MCS) can be used to provide a bridge to recovery or advanced therapies. Intra-aortic balloon pumps are commonly used to provide support to an unstable HF patient. There are several newer MCS devices available for the end-stage patient. Although they all provide hemodynamic support for unstable HF patients, one should recognize that each device has its challenges and side effects. These devices should only be utilized in highly skilled facilities with well-trained support staff. Some of the more commonly used new devices are:

- Extracorporeal membrane oxygenation
- TandemHeart
- Impella
- Centrimag

CHRONIC HEART FAILURE

This section focuses on the management of patients with chronic HF in an outpatient setting. Most of the initial workup of HF patient is usually done on the initial presentation in a hospital setting. It is important to obtain the comprehensive record of the entire workup of the HF patient and to start an individual profile for each patient. Outpatient management of HF serves as a checkpoint to address etiology, medication/device optimization, symptoms, advance therapies, and palliative care.

Etiology

Management of HF patients in an outpatient setting begins with further narrowing down the differential diagnosis of HF etiology. This step ensures that all the reversible causes of HF have been investigated and either addressed or ruled out. Presence of coronary disease, resistant hypertension, substance abuse, thyroid abnormalities, arrhythmias, and exposure to toxins are a few common and possibly reversible causes of HF. This information is key in tailoring the outpatient treatment to individual HF patients and improving outcomes.

Medication Optimization

Management of HF medications is a challenging yet critical step in the outpatient setting. In patients with HFrEF, every effort should be made to include BBs, ACE inhibitors, and aldosterone antagonists as part of medical therapy for chronic HF. The doses of these medications should be titrated up as tolerated by patients (see **Table 1**). Additional medical therapy such as hydralazine/nitrates combination, digoxin, and diuretics should also be initiated and maintained if the HF patient continues to be symptomatic or struggles with volume overload. ARBs should be used in HF patients who are ACE intolerant.

Volume Status and Symptom Surveillance

Monitoring the volume status of HF patients in an outpatient setting using physical examination (JVP, weight, edema), laboratory tests (BNP, sodium), and devices is crucial in maintaining overall quality of life and avoiding hospitalization. HF patients should be advised to monitor their daily weights and report any sudden significant changes (>2 lb/d or >5 lb/wk) to their HF care provider.[28] The diuretic therapy can be adjusted accordingly.

New York Heart Association (NYHA) functional classification is a simple and robust way of monitoring patients' symptoms in an outpatient setting. The clinician's goal is to get the HF patient to Class I or II functional class, and escalate the level of care in functional classes III and IV.

Device Optimization

Cardiac devices such as an implantable cardioverter-defibrillator (ICD), or cardiac resynchronization therapy (CRT) are now widely used in HFrEF patients who meet the appropriate criteria. As part of the evaluation of HF patients in an outpatient setting, the clinician should address the patient's candidacy for device therapy. In general, HFrEF patients with an ejection fraction of less than 35% who are optimized on medical therapy more than 3 to 6 months should be considered for ICD implantation. Patients with an ejection fraction of less than 35% because of acute myocardial infarction should wait for 40 days before ICD implantation.[29–31] ICDs should be reserved for patients with a reasonable expectation of survival in 1 year and adequate quality of life.

Patients with HFrEF and wide QRS morphology (ideally left bundle morphology with QRS >150 milliseconds) should be referred for CRT evaluation. Persistent right ventricular pacing caused by atrioventricular block or atrial fibrillation with slow ventricular response are also indications for CRT in HFrEF patients.

Referral to Advance Heart Failure Program

Despite optimal medical therapy, revascularization, and device therapies, a percentage of HF patients will progress to more advanced stages of the disease. The transition of an HF patient from stable on medical therapy to an advanced stage requiring MCS or heart transplantation can be subtle. Clinical findings that should trigger a referral to an advanced HF program include:

- Persistent NYHA class III to IV despite medical/device therapy
- Deteriorating renal or liver function (BUN >40 mg/dL or creatinine >1.8 mg/dL)
- BB or ACE-inhibitor intolerance owing to hypotension
- Increasing diuretic requirements (>120 mg/d or equivalent)
- Recurrent hospitalizations for HF (>1 in 6 months)

It is imperative to realize that once the patient develops irreversible organ damage, advanced therapies such as heart transplantation and LVADs may no longer be options. Therefore, timely referral to an HF program is important.

Hospice

As mentioned at the beginning of this article, there are more than 5 million patients who suffer from HF. Approximately 5% of the HF patient population is classified as NYHA IV, stage D. A small proportion of the NYHA IV patients will receive a heart transplant or LVAD therapy, but most of them will not be candidates for advanced therapies, with very poor outcomes (**Fig. 2**). Patients with end-stage HF have recurrent hospitalizations, deteriorating renal function, and poor quality of life. The patients and their caregivers are also burdened with significant physical and emotional stress in the final months of life.[31] Because the trajectory of end-stage HF is well known and documented, it is imperative for the physician to recognize and address such situations. Listed here are some of the signs that should prompt the clinician to start the end-of-life discussion with the patient and their family.

- NYHA IV symptoms despite optimal medical, surgical, and device therapies
- Deemed a poor candidate for transplant or LVAD
- Recurrent hospitalizations despite good compliance

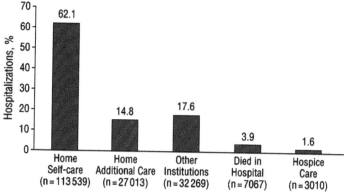

Fig. 2. Hospital discharge status of patients in the Acute Decompensated Heart Failure Registry (ADHERE) database. (*From* Hauptman PJ, Goodlin SJ, Lopatin M, et al. Characteristics of patients hospitalized with acute decompensated heart failure who are referred for hospice care. Arch Intern Med 2007;167(18):1990–97; with permission.)

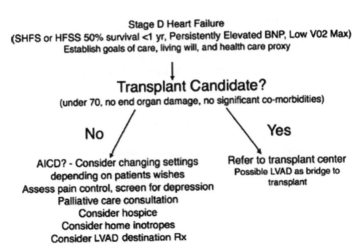

Stage D Heart Failure
(SHFS or HFSS 50% survival <1 yr, Persistently Elevated BNP, Low VO2 Max)
Establish goals of care, living will, and health care proxy

Transplant Candidate?
(under 70, no end organ damage, no significant co-morbidities)

No / Yes

AICD? - Consider changing settings
depending on patients wishes
Assess pain control, screen for depression
Palliative care consultation
Consider hospice
Consider home inotropes
Consider LVAD destination Rx

Refer to transplant center
Possible LVAD as bridge to
transplant

Fig. 3. Sample algorithm for treatment of end-stage heart failure. Prognostic scores are used to help evaluate which patients with optimally treated heart failure have stage D disease. Goals of care should be established in all patients. Appropriate patients should be referred for transplant/LVAD centers for evaluation. Pain should be addressed at every visit. Palliative care consultation, hospice care, or both may be considered. AICD, automated implanted cardioverter-defibrillator; BNP, B-type natriuretic peptide; HFSS, Heart Failure Survival Score; LVAD, left ventricular assist device; Rx, therapy; SHFS, Seattle Heart Failure Score; VO2 max, maximum oxygen uptake. (*From* Adler ED, Goldfinger JZ, Kalman J, et al. Palliative care in the treatment of advanced heart failure. Circulation 2009;120:2597–606; with permission.)

- Persistent ventricular arrhythmias despite medical and surgical interventions
- Profound cardiac cachexia

End-of-life discussions are always difficult, for both the patient and clinician. The primary physician's role is crucial in approaching the end-stage patient, as he or she usually has a closer and longer bond with the patient and family. Some of the common symptoms of end-stage HF are dyspnea, fatigue, pain, anorexia, and cachexia. Management of the HF patient in the palliative care and hospice stage focuses on patient comfort and quality of life.

Dyspnea can be treated with continuous infusion of home inotropes. Nitrates, opioids, and home oxygen are also effective in alleviating breathlessness. Caffeine and certain stimulants have been used to address fatigue in specific HF patients. Titrating down the dosage of BBs and ACE inhibitors, or stopping a class of medication altogether, can also be considered in hypotensive patients.

End-stage HF patients are prone to tachyarrhythmias and recurrent ICD shocks. ICD therapy should also be discussed with the patient and family. Discontinuing the defibrillating capability of the ICDs is a reasonable approach, although the CRT portion of the devices should be continued because it may provide relief of symptoms (**Fig. 3**).

REFERENCES

1. Giamouzis G, Kalogeropoulos A, Georgiopoulou V, et al. Hospitalization epidemic in patients with heart failure: risk factors, risk prediction, knowledge gaps, and future directions. J Card Fail 2011;17:54–75.

2. Fang J, Mensah GA, Croft JB, et al. Heart failure-related hospitalization in the U.S., 1979 to 2004. J Am Coll Cardiol 2008;52:428–34.
3. Nohria A, Mielniczuk LM, Stevenson LW. Evaluation and monitoring of patients with acute heart failure syndromes. Am J Cardiol 2005;96(6A):32G–40G.
4. Januzzi JL Jr, Sakhuja R, O'donoghue M, et al. Utility of amino-terminal pro-brain natriuretic peptide testing for prediction of 1-year mortality in patients with dyspnea treated in the emergency department. Arch Intern Med 2006;166:315–20.
5. Januzzi JL Jr, Rehman S, Mueller T, et al. Importance of biomarkers for long-term mortality prediction in acutely dyspneic patients. Clin Chem 2010;56:1814–21.
6. Horwich TB, Patel J, MacLellan WR, et al. Cardiac troponin I is associated with impaired hemodynamics, progressive left ventricular dysfunction, and increased mortality rates in advanced heart failure. Circulation 2003;108:833–8.
7. Rosenberg J, Gustafsson F, Galatius S, et al. Combination therapy with metolazone and loop diuretics in outpatients with refractory heart failure: an observational study and review of the literature. Cardiovasc Drugs Ther 2005;19:301–6.
8. Salvador DR, Rey NR, Ramos GC, et al. Continuous infusion versus bolus injection of loop diuretics in congestive heart failure. Cochrane Database Syst Rev 2005;(3):CD003178.
9. Publication Committee for the VMAC Investigators (Vasodilatation in the Management of Acute CHF). Intravenous nesiritide vs nitroglycerin for treatment of decompensated congestive heart failure: a randomized controlled trial. JAMA 2002;287:1531–40.
10. Cioffi G, Stefenelli C, Tarantini L, et al. Hemodynamic response to intensive unloading therapy (furosemide and nitroprusside) in patients >70 years of age with left ventricular systolic dysfunction and decompensated chronic heart failure. Am J Cardiol 2003;92:1050–6.
11. Colucci WS, Elkayam U, Horton DP, et al. Intravenous nesiritide, a natriuretic peptide, in the treatment of decompensated congestive heart failure. Nesiritide Study Group. N Engl J Med 2000;343:246–53.
12. Butler J, Young JB, Abraham WT, et al. Beta-blocker use and outcomes among hospitalized heart failure patients. J Am Coll Cardiol 2006;47:2462–9.
13. Beta-Blocker Evaluation of Survival Trial Investigators. A trial of the beta-blocker bucindolol in patients with advanced chronic heart failure. N Engl J Med 2001;344:1659–67.
14. Effects of carvedilol, a vasodilator-beta-blocker, in patients with congestive heart failure due to ischemic heart disease. Australia-New Zealand Heart Failure Research Collaborative Group. Circulation 1995;92:212–8.
15. Fonarow GC, Abraham WT, Albert NM, et al. Influence of beta-blocker continuation or withdrawal on outcomes in patients hospitalized with heart failure: findings from the OPTIMIZE-HF program. J Am Coll Cardiol 2008;52:190–9.
16. Effects of enalapril on mortality in severe congestive heart failure. Results of the Cooperative North Scandinavian Enalapril Survival Study (CONSENSUS). The CONSENSUS Trial Study Group. N Engl J Med 1987;316:1429–35.
17. Kober L, Torp-Pedersen C, Carlsen JE, et al. A clinical trial of the angiotensin-converting-enzyme inhibitor trandolapril in patients with left ventricular dysfunction after myocardial infarction. Trandolapril Cardiac Evaluation (TRACE) Study Group. N Engl J Med 1995;333:1670–6.
18. Cohn JN, Tognoni G. A randomized trial of the angiotensin-receptor blocker valsartan in chronic heart failure. N Engl J Med 2001;345:1667–75.
19. McMurray JJ, Ostergren J, Swedberg K, et al. Effects of candesartan in patients with chronic heart failure and reduced left-ventricular systolic function taking

angiotensin-converting-enzyme inhibitors: the CHARM-Added trial. Lancet 2003; 362:767–71.

20. Granger CB, McMurray JJ, Yusuf S, et al. Effects of candesartan in patients with chronic heart failure and reduced left-ventricular systolic function intolerant to angiotensin-converting-enzyme inhibitors: the CHARM-Alternative trial. Lancet 2003;362:772–6.

21. Pitt B, Remme W, Zannad F, et al. Eplerenone, a selective aldosterone blocker, in patients with left ventricular dysfunction after myocardial infarction. N Engl J Med 2003;348:1309–21.

22. Butler J, Ezekowitz JA, Collins SP, et al. Update on aldosterone antagonists use in heart failure with reduced left ventricular ejection fraction. Heart Failure Society of America Guidelines Committee. J Card Fail 2012;18:265–81.

23. Taylor AL, Ziesche S, Yancy C, et al. Combination of isosorbide dinitrate and hydralazine in blacks with heart failure. N Engl J Med 2004;351:2049–57.

24. The Digitalis Investigation Group. The effect of digoxin on mortality and morbidity in patients with heart failure. N Engl J Med 1997;336:525–33.

25. Klein L, O'Connor CM, Leimberger JD, et al. Lower serum sodium is associated with increased short-term mortality in hospitalized patients with worsening heart failure: results from the Outcomes of a Prospective Trial of Intravenous Milrinone for Exacerbations of Chronic Heart Failure (OPTIME-CHF) study. Circulation 2005;111:2454–60.

26. Aranda JM Jr, Schofield RS, Pauly DF, et al. Comparison of dobutamine versus milrinone therapy in hospitalized patients awaiting cardiac transplantation: a prospective, randomized trial. Am Heart J 2003;145:324–9.

27. Gorodeski EZ, Chu EC, Reese JR, et al. Prognosis on chronic dobutamine or milrinone infusions for stage D heart failure. Circ Heart Fail 2009;2:320–4.

28. Abraham WT, Compton S, Haas G, et al. Intrathoracic impedance vs daily weight monitoring for predicting worsening heart failure events: results of the Fluid Accumulation Status Trial (FAST). Congest Heart Fail 2011;17:51–5.

29. Zareba W, Piotrowicz K, McNitt S, et al. Implantable cardioverter-defibrillator efficacy in patients with heart failure and left ventricular dysfunction (from the MADIT II population). Am J Cardiol 2005;95:1487–91.

30. Barsheshet A, Wang PJ, Moss AJ, et al. Reverse remodeling and the risk of ventricular tachyarrhythmias in the MADIT-CRT (Multicenter Automatic Defibrillator Implantation Trial-Cardiac Resynchronization Therapy). J Am Coll Cardiol 2011; 57:2416–23.

31. Cleland JG, Ghosh J, Freemantle N, et al. Clinical trials update and cumulative meta-analyses from the American College of Cardiology: WATCH, SCD-HeFT, DINAMIT, CASINO, INSPIRE, STRATUS-US, RIO-Lipids and cardiac resynchronisation therapy in heart failure. Eur J Heart Fail 2004;6:501–8.

Emerging Role of Digital Technology and Remote Monitoring in the Care of Cardiac Patients

CrossMark

Javier E. Banchs, MD, FHRS[a],*, David Lee Scher, MD, FHRS[b]

KEYWORDS

• Arrhythmias • Heart failure • Implantable devices • Monitoring • Technology

KEY POINTS

• Advances in cardiac monitoring have resulted in higher diagnostic yields in patients presenting with clinical symptoms or consequences of cardiac arrhythmias.
• Advances in technology and communications have made possible effective remote monitoring of patients with cardiovascular diseases.
• Remote monitoring and telemonitoring has resulted in better outcomes among patients with implantable devices, but more evidence is needed to expand its application in other patient populations.

INTRODUCTION

Over the past 2 decades, advancements in digital technologies and mobile connectivity have led to the development of a variety of novel mobile and implantable devices with wireless capabilities. Many advances have occurred in cardiac telemetry and remote monitoring, cardiac implantable electronic devices (CIEDs), neurostimulators, and insulin pumps, among others. Widespread adoption of many of these devices and resources has led to improved quality of life and survival in affected patient populations.[1–9]

Heart disease remains the leading cause of death in the United States.[10] Despite progressive decline in deaths due to coronary artery disease and acute myocardial infarction attributed to the combination of public awareness, early treatment, and aggressive preventive strategies, a large percentage of health care spending is devoted to the management of patients with heart disease.[11] Chronic cardiac

[a] Department of Medicine, Division of Cardiology, Section of Cardiac Electrophysiology and Pacing, 2401 South 31st Street, Temple, TX 76508, USA; [b] Department of Medicine, Division of Cardiology, Penn State Hershey Heart & Vascular Institute, 500 University Drive, H047, Hershey, PA 17033, USA
* Corresponding author.
E-mail address: jbanchs@sw.org

Med Clin N Am 99 (2015) 877–896
http://dx.doi.org/10.1016/j.mcna.2015.02.013
0025-7125/15/$ – see front matter © 2015 Elsevier Inc. All rights reserved.

conditions including congestive heart failure (CHF) and cardiac arrhythmias are among the top 5 leading causes of hospital admissions in the United States.[12,13] The cost of care for patients with CHF in the United States is estimated at US $32 billion a year.[14]

This article describes the emerging role of digital technologies and remote monitoring in the management of patients with cardiovascular diseases. As a consequence of the rapid expansion of the field and its overlap with the exploding industry of consumer electronics, personal health, and fitness, the authors do not intend for this review to be all-inclusive.

MANAGEMENT GOALS

Digital technologies in cardiovascular diseases could be classified as preventive, diagnostic, and therapeutic. Opportunities for proof of concept include clinical benefit, safety, reliability, cost-effectiveness, adoption, and adherence rates. Like any other medical intervention, diagnostic or therapeutic new technology would be expected by the health care provider community to have undergone clinical trials with both clinical and nonclinical end points.

AVAILABLE TECHNOLOGIES
Wearable and Implantable Cardiac Rhythm Monitors

Diagnosis and management of the cardiac patient often requires ambulatory cardiac rhythm monitoring. A normal electrocardiogram at a given time does not exclude a cardiac arrhythmia associated with intermittent symptoms. Subclinical atrial fibrillation and ventricular tachycardia have significant prognostic implications.[15–21]

The Holter monitor has remained the most common tool used for ambulatory cardiac monitoring. The recording time (24 or 48 hours) and therefore the clinical utility of this device is limited. Obviously, if no subclinical abnormality or clinical event occurs during the recording period, the test result is indeterminate. In fact, the yield for symptoms such as palpitations, dizziness, chest pain, and syncope is low.[22–24] Advances in ambulatory heart rhythm monitoring include the external event recorder, with and without loop memory; the autotrigger feature; implantable loop recorder (ILR); mobile cardiac telemetry (MCT) originally introduced by CardioNet Inc (Malvern, PA, USA) as mobile cardiac outpatient telemetry (MCOT); heart cards and patch monitors; wearable pulse sensors; or smartphone-based rate and rhythm monitors. The appropriate device is chosen based on symptom frequency, patient health literacy, lifestyle, cost, and insurance coverage.[25,26]

The external event recorder only saves (for subsequent analysis) tracings, which are activated by the patient. The loop recorder, which is the most commonly used event monitor, saves a recording corresponding to the event and a period before and after. The corresponding signals can be transmitted over the telephone for analysis after the event. These monitors can be used for 7 to 21 days and are indicated for symptoms with a frequency greater than 24 to 48 hours. The autotrigger event recorder incorporates software that automatically identifies low, fast, and irregular heart rhythms.

The heart card is a more convenient portable cardiac rhythm recorder that can be carried for extended periods, stored in a wallet or pocket, and accessed at the time of symptoms. This device does not require skin electrodes (which could cause skin irritation in a few patients) or the inconvenient connector wires. The heart card has 2 spaced electrodes on the surface with a flat thin electrocardiographic recorder and transmitter. Placing the card on the skin against the chest during symptoms allows the patient to record a rhythm strip, which can then be transmitted over the telephone to the monitoring facility. This device requires that the symptom be long enough to be accessed and transmitted. Event recorders do not provide trends but rather symptom-driven snapshots; they have provide higher diagnostic yield than the Holter monitor.[27–31]

Advances in cellular communication technology, limitations of existing monitors, and the increasing demand for earlier and accurate diagnosis of cardiac arrhythmias led to the development of MCT systems. Multiple private providers offer MCT services with few variations. A set of electrodes and a cellular communication device is applied to the patient for 2 to 4 weeks for continuous monitoring. The signals are transmitted to a central station automatically when prespecified criteria for abnormalities are met or after manual patient activation in response to symptoms. Using cellular technology, the recordings are sent to live operators in real time and subsequently transmitted to the prescribing physician. MCT requires electrodes to be attached to the patient but provides continuous monitoring for up to a month, with a higher diagnostic yield when compared with traditional monitors. Most MCT services provide a 2-way text communication with the patient using the screen of the transmitter device and analysis of trends of arrhythmia and heart rate, useful for evaluation of ongoing therapy (**Fig. 1**). MCT is superior in outpatient diagnosis of symptoms that suggests arrhythmia and is effective in detecting atrial fibrillation in patients presenting with a cryptogenic stroke or after ablation for atrial fibrillation (**Table 1**).[32–36]

A newer generation of more comfortable and easier-to-use monitors placed on the skin via sticky patch allow for continuous cardiac rhythm recording of periods of up to 14 days (**Fig. 2**). At present, 2 of these devices are available in the United States. The Nuvant MCT (Corventis Inc, San Jose, CA, USA) acquired and rebranded as SEEQ by Medtronic, Inc, Minneapolis, MN, USA, is a patch MCT monitor. The Zio XT patch (iRhythm Technologies Inc, San Fransisco, CA, USA) is a 2-week continuous Holter monitor processed after it is returned by mail.[37–41] Both devices have a patient activation trigger for registration of clinical events. In general, longer periods of monitoring result in higher diagnostic yield.[27–31,42]

For patients with rather infrequent but clinically significant events such as syncope, suspected atrial fibrillation, long-term rhythm monitoring after cryptogenic stroke, or follow-up after suppressive therapy for cardiac arrhythmias, the ILR may be a more appropriate monitoring tool. The ILR is a small thin device with electrodes on the casing and wireless capabilities implanted in the subcutaneous tissue of the chest wall. The ILR automatically detects and records slow, fast, and irregular rhythms, or could be activated by an external remote control to record as a loop event recorder. Several events can be saved before transmission. Software in the device allows programming automatic detection alerts. Two brands of ILRs are available in the United States, SJM Confirm Implantable Cardiac Monitor (St. Jude Medical Inc, St Paul, MN, USA) and Reveal LINQ Insertable Cardiac Monitor (Medtronic, Inc) whose profile allows for it to be injectable at implant. Using the available wireless platform and battery technology of predecessor pacemakers and defibrillators, the ILR lasts for up to 3 years and can be interrogated remotely. Alerts are sent wirelessly automatically when the patient is in proximity to the transmitter. This technology is more expensive than traditional external monitors, which also permit multiple uses. Nevertheless, ILRs have become routine in the assessment of patients with cryptogenic stroke, unexplained syncope, and rare but significant symptoms, and for selected follow-up after therapeutic arrhythmia interventions. ILRs are preferred in these clinical scenarios because of their long battery life, remote capabilities, and simplicity of use despite requiring implantation (**Fig. 3**).[15,43–51]

A variety of personal heart rate monitors are available as part of nonprescription multipurpose consumer products and used for detection of arrhythmias, including automatic

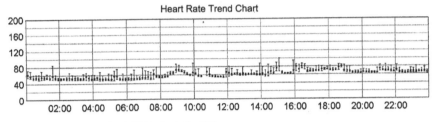

CARDIONET

Mobile Cardiac Outpatient Telemetry (MCOT)
(TEL) 866-426-4401 (FAX) 866-426-4403

Daily Patient Report

Report ID:

Patient Name:		Prescribing Physician:
Date of Birth:	Gender:	Scott & White
Patient Phone:		2401 South 31st St.
Patient ID:		Temple, TX 76508
Medical Record:		
Enrollment:		

Diagnosis (ICD9): 780.2 Syncope and collapse

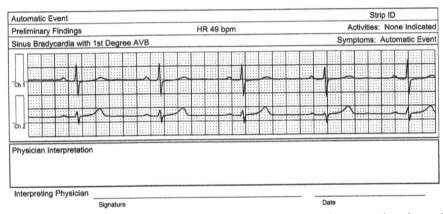

Heart Rate Trend Chart

* Heart rate cannot be calculated due to excessive artifact.

Automatic Event		Strip ID
Preliminary Findings	HR 49 bpm	Activities: None Indicated
Sinus Bradycardia with 1st Degree AVB		Symptoms: Automatic Event

Physician Interpretation

Interpreting Physician _____   Date _____
Signature

Fig. 1. MCOT daily report. MCOT provides continuous outpatient telemetry and can be used for up to 30 days. A daily report with heart rate trends and a strip sample is generated. Automatically detected arrhythmias and patient-triggered events are documented and correlated with electrocardiographic findings in real time. Patient identifiers and dates have been removed. (*Courtesy of* CardioNet, Malvern, PA; with permission.)

blood pressure (BP) cuffs with heart rate readings.[52–54] Some of these have been validated against electrocardiographic recordings in their accuracy of detecting heart rate variability.[55,56] Portable pulse oximeters also assess heart rate. Many of these personal devices are now available with memory or connectivity to personal computers, tablets, or smartphones for storage, trending, or communication of the data.

Remote Monitoring of Pacemakers, Defibrillators, and Implantable Pressure Sensors

CIEDs, which include pacemakers and implantable cardioverter-defibrillators (ICDs), have had wireless remote monitoring capabilities since 2000 (**Figs. 4** and **5**). Remote monitoring of CIEDs was first introduced as a potential revenue stream. However, after an ICD lead defect was first diagnosed via crowd-sourced data prompting an advisory and subsequently a recall, the Heart Rhythm Society adopted it as a standard of care for the postimplant follow-up of CIEDs.[57]

Most CIEDs, including some ILRs, can alert the health care team in charge of follow-up of the occurrence of atrial fibrillation, ventricular arrhythmias, device therapies, lead failure, electromagnetic interference, patient activity, and battery depletion, among other parameters, before a scheduled follow-up and frequently with the patient asymptomatic. Early detection of atrial fibrillation or ventricular arrhythmias could lead to early intervention and potential prevention of stroke, heart failure exacerbation, or ICD shocks (**Fig. 6**).[58–63] Device-based remote monitoring can also identify the need for upgrading a pacemaker to an ICD (for prevention of sudden death), ischemia assessment, catheter ablation of arrhythmia, or optimization of medical therapy.[64–66] The prompt identification of lead failure and supraventricular arrhythmias plays an important role in the prevention of inappropriate ICD shocks, which are known to be associated with high morbidity and mortality.[67,68]

The feasibility and benefit of remote monitoring of CIEDs have been shown in several clinical trials to be comparable, and in some cases superior, to in-person follow-up, resulting in shorter occurrence to intervention time for detected arrhythmias or device function problems. The Lumos-T Safely Reduces Routine Office Device Follow-Up (TRUST) was a prospective, randomized, multicenter trial of 1339 patients with ICDs, randomized 2:1 to remote monitoring or conventional follow-up. Home monitoring resulted in a 45% reduction of in-hospital evaluations without compromising safety and led to significantly shorter intervention time in response to arrhythmic events (<2 days vs 36 days in the conventional group).[58] The ALTITUDE survival study evaluated outcomes in a large population of patients with ICD and cardiac resynchronization therapy (CRT). This trial involved prospective, nonrandomized clinical data collection. Events and survival data from 185,778 patients were analyzed comparing patients followed up in device clinics with those followed up remotely. Survival up to 5 years among the 69,556 patients followed up remotely was higher than that in the 116,222 individuals followed up in device clinics, corresponding to a 50% relative risk reduction in mortality.[59] The Clinical Evaluation of Remote Notification to Reduce Time to Clinical Decision (CONNECT) trial was a prospective, randomized, multicenter clinical trial of 1997 patients receiving ICDs and CRT defibrillators followed up for 15 months. Individuals were randomized 1:1 to remote monitoring or in-office follow-up. There was significant reduction in time to response to clinical events (4.6 vs 22 days) and a shorter length of stay for cardiovascular hospitalizations (3.3 vs 4 days) for patients followed up remotely compared with the control group.[60]

Other studies, including the pacemaker randomized trials PREFER (Pacemaker Remote Follow-up Evaluation and Review) (897 patients)[62] and COMPAS (COMPArative follow-up Schedule with home monitoring) (538 patients)[63] and a more recent ICD trial ECOST (Effectiveness and Cost of ICDs Follow-up Schedule with Telecardiology) (433 patients),[61] showed similar benefits of remote monitoring, including a shorter time to diagnosis of clinical events,[62] fewer hospitalizations for atrial arrhythmias and strokes, less clinic visits,[63] noninferiority with respect to major adverse events, lower incidence of all ICD shocks, inappropriate shocks, and longer battery longevity.[61]

Sensors enhance CIED remote monitoring and diagnostic capabilities. Motion sensors in the form of accelerometers, piezoelectric crystals, or blended sensors are the standard of care for effective pacing rate adjustments according to physical activity.[69] Similarly, some devices use adjuvant changes in transthoracic impedance measurements to further adjust pacing rates.[70] Impedance changes within the lead electrodes have been used as surrogate changes in autonomic tone.[71,72]

Table 1
Comparison of published data on diagnostic yields of different ambulatory cardiac rhythm monitoring devices

Reference	Device	Period	Condition	Patients	Yield	Results
Zeldis et al,[22] 1980	Holter	24 h	Palpitations, dyspnea, chest discomfort, dizziness, and syncope	518	10%	Presenting symptoms corresponded with normal recording in 126 (24%) and with arrhythmia in 50 (10%) patients
Gibson & Heitzman,[23] 1984	Holter	24 h	Syncope	1512	2%	Syncope in 15 patients (7 with arrhythmia), 0.4% Presyncope in 241 patients (24 with arrhythmia), 1.6%
Bass et al,[24] 1990	Holter	24–72 h	Syncope	95	27% (72 h)	In the first 24 h, Holter identified arrhythmia in 15%; in the second 24 h, additional 9%; and in the third, 3%
Linzer et al,[27] 1990	ERec 1 mo	Up to 1 mo	Syncope	54	25%	Prior negative result on Holter; 14 of 57 patients were found to have an arrhythmia
Kinlay et al,[28] 1996	Holter vs ERec	48 h vs up to 3 mo	Palpitations	43	35% vs 67%[a]	Randomly assigned. ERec detected 8 clinically significant arrhythmias (19%), Holter none. P<.05
Fogel et al,[29] 1997	ERec	1 mo or more	Palpitations, presyncope, syncope	184	33%	Patients with heart disease underwent EP study; 33% had symptoms and documented arrhythmia; 22% has symptoms with no arrhythmia
Sivakumaran et al,[30] 2003	Holter vs ERec	48 h vs 1 mo	Syncope or presyncope	100	64% vs 24%[a]	Probability of symptom: arrhythmia correlation 22% for Holter and 56% for ERec; P<.0001

Study	Device/Comparison	Duration	Indication	N	Result	Comments
Reiffel et al,[31] 2005	Holter vs ERec vs autotriggered ERec	24 h vs 1 mo	Palpitations, syncope, dizziness, AF, dyspnea, chest pain, and arrhythmias	1800	6.2% vs 17% vs 36%	Retrospective database; the autotriggered ERec provided the higher yield of diagnostic events (36%); it was more effective in capturing asymptomatic AF (52 vs 1 with ERec)
Joshi et al,[32] 2005	MCOT	2–28 d	Palpitations, drug monitoring, dizziness, syncope, and arrhythmias	100	51%[b]	Initial experience of consecutive patients; clinically significant arrhythmia detected in 51%, asymptomatic in 25% of the entire population; 13% found to have asymptomatic AF
Rothman et al,[33] 2007	MCOT vs ERec	Up to 1 mo	Syncope, presyncope, and palpitations	266	88% vs 69%[a]	Randomized clinical trial; prior negative result on Holter; a diagnosis was made in 88% with MCOT vs 75% with ERec; $P = .008$ MCOT confirmed a significant clinical arrhythmia in 41% vs 15% in the ERec group; $P<.001$
Tayal et al,[34] 2008	MCOT	Up to 21 d	Cryptogenic stroke	56	23% AF[b]	Series of consecutive patients; 27 episodes of asymptomatic AF detected in 13 patients; 15% episodes lasted 4–24 h
Miller et al,[35] 2013	MCOT	Up to 30 d	Cryptogenic stroke	156	17% AF[b]	Retrospective study; rate of AF detection was 3.9% in 48 h, 9.2% in 7 d, 15.1% in 14 d, and 19.5% in 21 d

Abbreviations: AF, atrial fibrillation; EP, electrophysiology; ERec, Event Recorder.
[a] Includes exclusion of arrhythmia with symptoms during normal recording.
[b] Includes asymptomatic arrhythmias.
Data from Refs.[22–24,27–35]

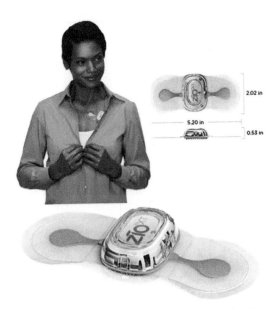

Fig. 2. Patch monitor. The Zio XT patch monitor is attached to the chest and could be used for up to 14 days. This monitor provides continuous cardiac rhythm monitoring and the ability of marking clinical events. After the patch is mailed back and processed, trends and electrocardiographic recordings are made available over the Internet in a secured Web site. (*Courtesy of* iRhythm Technologies, San Fransisco, CA; with permission.)

Variations in transthoracic impedance have been shown to correlate with variations in pulmonary congestion and are the basis of current heart failure monitoring algorithms of ICDs and CRT devices (**Fig. 7**).[73–75] Significant drops below a prespecified threshold are interpreted as impending heart failure, but despite reasonably good correlation between pulmonary congestion and measured transthoracic impedance, no significant impact in clinical outcomes has been demonstrated. Problems with false-positive results of measurements in patients with lung disease have been noted.

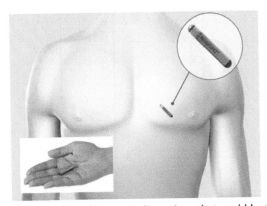

Fig. 3. Reveal LINQ is an ILR of small enough dimensions that could be injected through a small incision made with a cutting instrument. The battery life is at least 3 years, and it automatically detects atrial fibrillation and stores electrocardiographic recordings on patient activation. Using CareLink Network (Medtronic, Inc), the recorded information can be transmitted remotely. (Reproduced with permission of Medtronic, Inc.)

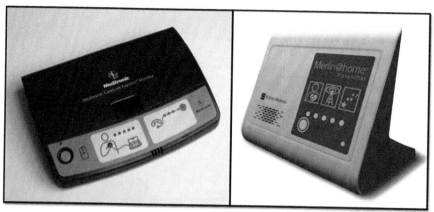

Fig. 4. Home monitor and transmitter units CareLink and Merlin@home (St. Jude Medical). The units are connected at home either to the home phone line or with a cellular adaptor and used for periodic wireless transmission of device data in the form of scheduled remote interrogation, patient-initiated transmission, or automatic alerts integrated to a device remote monitor program. (CareLink image reproduced with permission of Medtronic, Inc. Accent, Merlin@home, Potico and St. Jude Medical are trademarks of St. Jude Medical, Inc., or its related companies. Reprinted with permission of St. Jude Medical, © 2015. All rights reserved.)

Other means of predicting heart failure exacerbation and monitoring therapy involve direct measurements of right ventricular, pulmonary artery, or left atrial pressures with implantable sensors.[76–79] A prospective, randomized, single-blinded clinical trial telemonitoring right ventricular pressure in 274 patients with heart failure with such a system COMPASS-HF (Chronicle Offers Management to Patients with Advanced Signs and Symptoms of Heart Failure) met the safety end points but failed to meet the clinical end point of reduction in heart-failure-related events. Retrospectively, it demonstrated

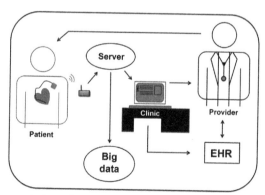

Fig. 5. Generic representation of a remote monitoring system for CIEDs. Information from the implanted device is received wirelessly by a home unit that via telephone (or cellular phone) sends the information to a network server to be downloaded via Internet in the device clinic. Transmissions are received as scheduled remote interrogation, patient-initiated transmission, or automatic alerts and communicated to the provider for decision making. When necessary the patient is contacted for the appropriate intervention. Data can be incorporated into the electronic health record (EHR) or used for analysis to identify trends and better define management protocols.

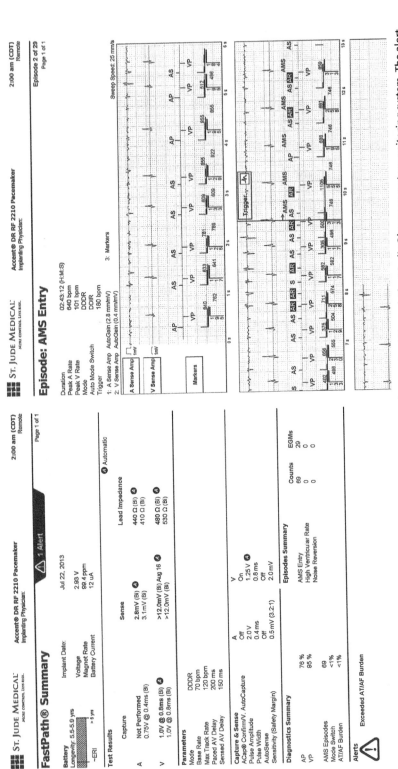

Fig. 6. Automatic alert report from a St. Jude Medical dual-chamber pacemaker received through the Merlin@home remote monitoring system. The alert corresponds to an episode of atrial fibrillation lasting 2 hours and 43 minutes. Details about battery life, automatic lead testing, and programmed parameters (*left panel*) and details of electrogram recordings from the atrial and ventricular leads are made available to the clinician (*right panel*) for management decision making regarding the underlying condition, recorded arrhythmias, or the device itself. Early identification of atrial fibrillation permits initiation of anticoagulation for stroke prevention in patients with subclinical atrial fibrillation. Patient identifiers and some dates have been removed (AMS, Auto Mode Switch). (Accent, Merlin@home, and St. Jude Medical are trademarks of St. Jude Medical, Inc., or its related companies. Reprinted with permission of St. Jude Medical. © 2015. All rights reserved.)

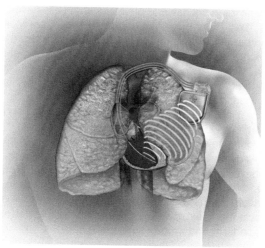

Fig. 7. Cartoon depicting the transthoracic impedance monitor system OptiVol (Medtronic, Inc) developed for early diagnosis of heart failure exacerbation. Changes of intrathoracic impedance correspond to pulmonary congestion and can be monitored remotely using the CareLink Network. Similar systems are also available from other CIED manufacturers. (Reproduced with permission of Medtronic, Inc.)

reduction in time to first heart failure hospitalization.[76] The LAPTOP-HF (Left Atrial Pressure Monitoring to Optimize Heart Failure Therapy) trial using an implantable sensor for direct monitoring of left atrial pressure is still ongoing,[79] but the Cardio-MEMS Heart Failure System (St. Jude Medical, Inc, St Paul, MN) implantable pulmonary artery pressure sensor received US Food and Drug Administration (FDA) approval for clinical use early in 2014 after showing a 39% reduction in hospital readmissions over 6 months, among 550 patients with New York Heart Association class III heart failure in the CHAMPION (CardioMEMS Heart Sensor Allows Monitoring of Pressure to Improve Outcomes in NYHA Class III Heart Failure Patients) trial.[77]

Electrocardiographic manifestations of ischemia can also be monitored continuously in the outpatient setting with implantable monitors. Stand-alone ST-segment elevation monitors and software incorporated into CIEDs for early diagnosis of acute coronary syndromes are currently undergoing evaluation in clinical trials.[80]

Despite favorable clinical data and demonstrated cost savings,[81,82] a study of 39,158 implanted devices showed that only 47% of patients activated remote monitoring, with significant variation among study sites.[83]

Other Digital Technology Tools

Outpatient management of the cardiac patient frequently involves assessment of symptoms and monitoring of other comorbid conditions such as diabetes and chronic obstructive pulmonary disease. Symptoms and glucose or BP diaries are commonly used in medical practice, but real-time data transmission has traditionally been difficult to impossible. New care models of patient engagement and shared decision making and the advent of mobile health technologies will soon transform today's practices. Even structured telephone-based monitoring programs facilitate this interaction and have shown the potential of significantly affecting clinical outcomes. Several studies have demonstrated higher reductions in BP among patients with hypertension using home BP monitoring systems with feedback and support.[84–86] Improvement of control of both glucose and lipid levels has also been reported among patients with diabetes.[87] Telephone interventions and postdischarge calls have been widely adopted for heart failure. The Trans-European Network-Home-Care Management System (TEN-HMS) study prospectively randomized 426 patients to usual care, telemonitoring, and nurse telephone support. The 1-year mortality rates were 45%, 29%, and 27%, respectively, but no significant differences in hospitalization rates was observed.[88] A recent meta-analysis of telemonitoring for heart failure found significant reduction in readmissions and cost of care.[89–91]

Additional resources include electronic medication packaging and medication message reminders using computer- or smartphone-based software.[92,93] One of the most promising sensor technologies is Proteus Digital's medication adherence tool (Proteus Digital Health, Inc, Redwood City, CA, USA); it is a physiologic sensor placed on a pill, which, when activated by gastric acid, emits a signal to a skin patch electrode that sends vital sign information and documents ingestion of the said pill. Smartphones and tablets, with consumer-directed wellness apps (tracking activity, heart rates, and sleep) have recently gained popularity.[94] Text messaging has been implemented as a tool for managing hypertension and obesity and supporting smoking cessation interventions.[95–98] A survey of 118 cardiac patients revealed that 85% own a computer, tablet, or similar device; 83% own a cell phone, 75% use the e-mail; 55% use text messaging; close to half use apps; and 32% of use health-related apps.[99] These resources have a great potential to affect health care delivery and its outcomes.

FUTURE CONSIDERATIONS

Mobile technology is an area of rapid expansion. Cellular phones have evolved from the concept of a mobile telephone to a fully operational handheld computer equipped with sensors and highly efficient connectivity; 53% of cell phone owners have a smartphone.[94] Software applications (apps) with specific functions and Internet support are being developed at a very fast pace to support needs in all aspects of life including health care. Apps to support and track exercise are available for different disciplines, providing routines, coaching with voice and video, links to specific products, caloric expenditure calculation, geolocation, covered distance, as well as time and data trends. Nutrition information, caloric information of food, calorie count and balance, as well as links to recipes and products are also available. The high resolution of the cameras available today in smartphones permits the detection of minimal changes in skin color and body parts motion caused by pulsatile blood flow and respiration, which has made possible the development of apps that can measure heart and respiratory rate reliably.[100–102] AliveCor Heart Monitor (AliveCor, Inc, San Francisco, CA, USA) is a Bluetooth-enabled electrocardiographic monitor that connects with an app in a smartphone for a single-lead rhythm recording. The recording can be stored and submitted for real-time professional interpretation. The device has recently been approved by the FDA for its algorithmic identification of atrial fibrillation.[103,104] The development of smaller and more accurate sensors, integrated with the computing power, data storage, and transfer capabilities of current personal handheld communication devices, holds the promise of very powerful diagnostic and monitoring tools (**Fig. 8**). Other sensors can now be placed on skin for monitoring or as part of transdermal drug delivery systems with feedback loops.[105]

Telehealth and remote monitoring are solutions to physician shortages, both national and regional.[106] Sensors can be divided into vital sign sensors, activities-of-daily-living sensors, and home sensors. An example of an integrated sensing system is GrandCare Systems (West Bend, WI).

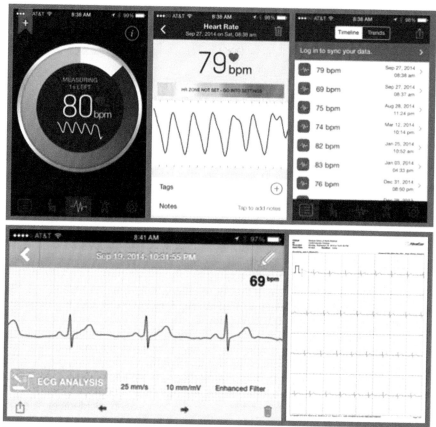

Fig. 8. Smartphone-based mobile cardiac monitoring applications. Top panel corresponds to screen images of an instant heart rate application for smartphones that uses the light and camera of the device to measure heart rate based on pulsatile skin color changes (*left*). Information regarding the time and circumstances of the measurement can be documented (*center*) and trends of heart rate are available for storage and communication (*right*). The bottom panel corresponds to a screen image of a cardiac rhythm recording performed with the AliveCor device on a smartphone (*left*), which could also be stored, submitted for professional analysis, or saved as a pdf document for printing or sharing electronically (*right*).

Development of technology and devices in health care encounters the obvious challenges of research and development. Safety and effectiveness must be demonstrated for FDA approval for what the FDA defines as medical devices. This fact is not true of the vast majority of health and wellness apps as per the FDA Guidance of Mobile Medical Applications (which do not fall under the definition of a medical device), and their safety, efficacy, and privacy are left up to the developer and user. Evidence of positive clinical or economic outcomes is required for their acceptance. Cost and reimbursement become the next decisive factors for their widespread adoption.

SUMMARY

Remote patient monitoring, mobile apps, and wireless sensors are in relatively early stages of development and adoption. However, the "perfect storm" of rapidly aging populations, unsustainable health care expenditures, and rapid uptake of mobile technologies have created fertile ground for adoption. Digital technologies are expected to become critical elements of diagnosis, long-term disease management, and patient engagement.

REFERENCES

1. González-Molero I, Domínguez-López M, Guerrero M, et al. Use of telemedicine in subjects with type 1 diabetes equipped with an insulin pump and real-time continuous glucose monitoring. J Telemed Telecare 2012;18(6):328–32.
2. Müller-Godeffroy E, Treichel S, Wagner VM, German Working Group for Paediatric Pump Therapy. Investigation of quality of life and family burden issues during insulin pump therapy in children with Type 1 diabetes mellitus–a large-scale multicentre pilot study. Diabet Med 2009;26(5):493–501.
3. Wu C, Sharan AD. Neurostimulation for the treatment of epilepsy: a review of current surgical interventions. Neuromodulation 2013;16(1):10–24.
4. Devroede G, Giese C, Wexner SD, et al. Quality of life is markedly improved in patients with fecal incontinence after sacral nerve stimulation. Female Pelvic Med Reconstr Surg 2012;18(2):103–12.
5. Weaver FM, Follett K, Stern M, et al. Bilateral deep brain stimulation vs best medical therapy for patients with advanced Parkinson disease: a randomized controlled trial. JAMA 2009;301(1):63–73.
6. Chen S, Yin Y, Krucoff MW. Effect of cardiac resynchronization therapy and implantable cardioverter defibrillator on quality of life in patients with heart failure: a meta-analysis. Europace 2012;14(11):1602–7.
7. Bardy GH, Lee KL, Mark DB, et al. Amiodarone or an implantable cardioverter-defibrillator for congestive heart failure. N Engl J Med 2005;352:225–37.
8. Bristow MR, Saxon LA, Boehmer J, et al, Comparison of Medical Therapy, Pacing, and Defibrillation in Heart Failure (COMPANION) Investigators. Cardiac-resynchronization therapy with or without an implantable defibrillator in advanced chronic heart failure. N Engl J Med 2004;350(21):2140–50.
9. Moss AJ, Zareba W, Hall WJ, et al, Multicenter Automatic Defibrillator Implantation Trial II Investigators. Prophylactic implantation of a defibrillator in patients with myocardial infarction and reduced ejection fraction. N Engl J Med 2002;346(12):877–83.
10. Murphy SL, Xu JQ, Kochanek KD. Deaths: final data for 2010. Natl Vital Stat Rep 2013;61(4):1–117.
11. Go AS, Mozaffarian D, Roger VL, et al. Heart disease and stroke statistics - 2013 update: a report from the American Heart Association. Circulation 2013;127:e6–245.
12. Hines AL, Barrett ML, Jiang HJ, et al. Conditions with the largest number of adult hospital readmissions by payer, 2011. AHRQ Brief. 2014. Available at: http://www.hcup-us.ahrq.gov/reports/statbriefs/sb172-Conditions-Readmissions-Payer.pdf. Accessed September 6, 2014.
13. Desai AS, Stevenson LW. Special report: rehospitalization for heart failure: predict or prevent? Circulation 2012;126:501–6.
14. Heidenreich PA, Trogdon JG, Khavjou OA, et al. Forecasting the future of cardiovascular disease in the United States: a policy statement from the American Heart Association. Circulation 2011;123(8):933–44.
15. Sanna T, Diener HC, Passman RS, et al. Cryptogenic stroke and underlying atrial fibrillation. N Engl J Med 2014;370(26):2478–86.

16. Healey JS, Connolly SJ, Gold MR, et al. Subclinical atrial fibrillation and the risk of stroke. N Engl J Med 2012;366(2):120–9.

17. Friberg L, Hammar N, Rosenqvist M. Stroke in paroxysmal atrial fibrillation: report from the Stockholm Cohort of Atrial Fibrillation. Eur Heart J 2010;31(8): 967–75.

18. Wolf PA, Abbott RD, Kannel WB. Atrial fibrillation as an independent risk factor for stroke: the Framingham Study. Stroke 1991;22(8):983–8.

19. Marchlinski FE, Buxton AE, Flores BT, et al. Value of Holter monitoring in identifying risk for sustained ventricular arrhythmia recurrence on amiodarone. Am J Cardiol 1985;55(6):709–12.

20. Kowey PR, Waxman HL, Greenspon A, et al. Value of electrophysiologic testing in patients with previous myocardial infarction and nonsustained ventricular tachycardia. Philadelphia Arrhythmia Group. Am J Cardiol 1990;65(9):594–8.

21. Grimm W, Christ M, Maisch B. Long runs of non-sustained ventricular tachycardia on 24-hour ambulatory electrocardiogram predict major arrhythmic events in patients with idiopathic dilated cardiomyopathy. Pacing Clin Electrophysiol 2005;28(Suppl 1):S207–10.

22. Zeldis SM, Levine BJ, Michelson EL, et al. Cardiovascular complaints. Correlation with cardiac arrhythmias on 24-hour electrocardiographic monitoring. Chest 1980;78(3):456–61.

23. Gibson TC, Heitzman MR. Diagnostic efficacy of 24-hour electrocardiographic monitoring for syncope. Am J Cardiol 1984;53(8):1013–7.

24. Bass EB, Curtiss EI, Arena VC, et al. The duration of Holter monitoring in patients with syncope. Is 24 hours enough? Arch Intern Med 1990;150(5):1073–8.

25. Zimetbaum P, Goldman A. Ambulatory arrhythmia monitoring: choosing the right device. Circulation 2010;122:1629–36.

26. Zimetbaum P, Josephson ME. Evaluation of patients with palpitations. N Engl J Med 1998;338(19):1369–73.

27. Linzer M, Pritchett EL, Pontinen M, et al. Incremental diagnostic yield of loop electrocardiographic recorders in unexplained syncope. Am J Cardiol 1990; 66(2):214–9.

28. Kinlay S, Leitch JW, Neil A, et al. Cardiac event recorders yield more diagnoses and are more cost-effective than 48-hour Holter monitoring in patients with palpitations. A controlled clinical trial. Ann Intern Med 1996; 124(1 Pt 1):16–20.

29. Fogel RI, Evans JJ, Prystowsky EN. Utility and cost of event recorders in the diagnosis of palpitations, presyncope, and syncope. Am J Cardiol 1997;79(2): 207–8.

30. Sivakumaran S, Krahn AD, Klein GJ, et al. A prospective randomized comparison of loop recorders versus Holter monitors in patients with syncope or presyncope. Am J Med 2003;115(1):1–5.

31. Reiffel JA, Schwartzberg R, Murray M. Comparison of autotriggered memory loop recorders versus standard loop recorders versus 24-hour Holter monitors for arrhythmia detection. Am J Cardiol 2005;95:1055–9.

32. Joshi AK, Kowey PR, Prystowsky EN, et al. First experience with a Mobile Cardiac Outpatient Telemetry (MCOT) system for the diagnosis and management of cardiac arrhythmia. Am J Cardiol 2005;95(7):878–81.

33. Rothman SA, Laughlin JC, Seltzer J, et al. The diagnosis of cardiac arrhythmias: a prospective multi-center randomized study comparing mobile cardiac outpatient telemetry versus standard loop event monitoring. J Cardiovasc Electrophysiol 2007;18(3):241–7.

34. Tayal AH, Tian M, Kelly KM, et al. Atrial fibrillation detected by mobile cardiac outpatient telemetry in cryptogenic TIA or stroke. Neurology 2008;71(21):1696–701.

35. Miller DJ, Khan MA, Schultz LR, et al. Outpatient cardiac telemetry detects a high rate of atrial fibrillation in cryptogenic stroke. J Neurol Sci 2013;324(1–2): 57–61.

36. Vasamreddy CR, Dalal D, Dong J, et al. Symptomatic and asymptomatic atrial fibrillation in patients undergoing radiofrequency catheter ablation. J Cardiovasc Electrophysiol 2006;17(2):134–9.

37. Lobodzinski SS, Laks MM. New devices for very long-term ECG monitoring. Cardiol J 2012;19:210–4.

38. Engel JM, Chakravarthy N, Katra RP, et al. Estimation of patient compliance in application of adherent mobile cardiac telemetry device. Conf Proc IEEE Eng Med Biol Soc 2011;2011:1536–9.

39. Engel JM, Mehta V, Fogoros R, et al. Study of arrhythmia prevalence in NUVANT Mobile Cardiac Telemetry system patients. Conf Proc IEEE Eng Med Biol Soc 2012;2012:2440–3.

40. Turakhia MP, Hoang DD, Zimetbaum P, et al. Diagnostic utility of a novel leadless arrhythmia monitoring device. Am J Cardiol 2013;112(4):520–4.

41. Barrett PM, Komatireddy R, Haaser S, et al. Comparison of 24-hour Holter monitoring with 14-day novel adhesive patch electrocardiographic monitoring. Am J Med 2014;127(1):95.e11–7.

42. Assar MD, Krahn AD, Klein GJ, et al. Optimal duration of monitoring in patients with unexplained syncope. Am J Cardiol 2003;92(10):1231–3.

43. Cotter PE, Martin PJ, Ring L, et al. Incidence of atrial fibrillation detected by implantable loop recorders in unexplained stroke. Neurology 2013;80(17): 1546–50.

44. Mittal S, Pokushalov E, Romanov A, et al. Long-term ECG monitoring using an implantable loop recorder for the detection of atrial fibrillation after cavotricuspid isthmus ablation in patients with atrial flutter. Heart Rhythm 2013;10(11):1598–604.

45. Christensen LM, Krieger DW, Højberg S, et al. Paroxysmal atrial fibrillation occurs often in cryptogenic ischaemic stroke. Final results from the SURPRISE study. Eur J Neurol 2014;21(6):884–9.

46. Krahn AD, Klein GJ, Yee R, et al. Use of an extended monitoring strategy in patients with problematic syncope. Reveal Investigators. Circulation 1999;99(3):406–10.

47. Zaidi A, Clough P, Cooper P, et al. Misdiagnosis of epilepsy: many seizure-like attacks have a cardiovascular cause. J Am Coll Cardiol 2000;36(1):181–4.

48. Seidl K, Rameken M, Breunung S, et al. Diagnostic assessment of recurrent unexplained syncope with a new subcutaneously implantable loop recorder. Reveal-Investigators. Europace 2000;2(3):256–62.

49. Krahn AD, Klein GJ, Yee R, et al. Randomized assessment of syncope trial: conventional diagnostic testing versus a prolonged monitoring strategy. Circulation 2001;104(1):46–51.

50. Giada F, Gulizia M, Francese M, et al. Recurrent unexplained palpitations (RUP) study comparison of implantable loop recorder versus conventional diagnostic strategy. J Am Coll Cardiol 2007;49(19):1951–6.

51. Kapa S, Epstein AE, Callans DJ, et al. Assessing arrhythmia burden after catheter ablation of atrial fibrillation using an implantable loop recorder: the ABACUS study. J Cardiovasc Electrophysiol 2013;24(8):875–81.

52. Munschauer FE 3rd, Sohocki D, Smith Carrow S, et al. A community education program on atrial fibrillation: implications of pulse self-examination on awareness and behavior. J Stroke Cerebrovasc Dis 2004;13(5):208–13.

53. Wiesel J, Abraham S, Messineo FC. Screening for asymptomatic atrial fibrillation while monitoring the blood pressure at home: trial of regular versus irregular pulse for prevention of stroke (TRIPPS 2.0). Am J Cardiol 2013;111(11): 1598–601.

54. Virtanen R, Kryssi V, Vasankari T, et al. Self-detection of atrial fibrillation in an aged population - The LietoAF Study. Eur J Prev Cardiol 2014;21:1437–42.

55. Gamelin FX, Berthoin S, Bosquet L. Validity of the polar S810 heart rate monitor to measure R-R intervals at rest. Med Sci Sports Exerc 2006;38(5):887–93.

56. Vanderlei LC, Silva RA, Pastre CM, et al. Comparison of the Polar S810i monitor and the ECG for the analysis of heart rate variability in the time and frequency domains. Braz J Med Biol Res 2008;41(10):854–9.

57. Wilkoff BL, Auricchio A, Brugada J, et al. HRS/EHRA expert consensus on the monitoring of cardiovascular implantable electronic devices (CIEDs): description of techniques, indications, personnel, frequency and ethical considerations. Heart Rhythm 2008;5(6):907–25.

58. Varma N, Epstein AE, Irimpen A, et al. Efficacy and safety of automatic remote monitoring for implantable cardioverter-defibrillator follow-up: the Lumos-T Safely Reduces Routine Office Device Follow-up (TRUST) trial. Circulation 2010;122(4):325–32.

59. Saxon LA, Hayes DL, Gilliam FR, et al. Long-term outcome after ICD and CRT implantation and influence of remote device follow-up: the ALTITUDE survival study. Circulation 2010;122(23):2359–67.

60. Crossley GH, Boyle A, Vitense H, et al. The CONNECT (Clinical Evaluation of Remote Notification to Reduce Time to Clinical Decision) trial: the value of wireless remote monitoring with automatic clinician alerts. J Am Coll Cardiol 2011; 57(10):1181–9.

61. Guédon-Moreau L, Lacroix D, Sadoul N, et al. A randomized study of remote follow-up of implantable cardioverter defibrillators: safety and efficacy report of the ECOST trial. Eur Heart J 2013;34(8):605–14.

62. Crossley GH, Chen J, Choucair W, et al. Clinical benefits of remote versus transtelephonic monitoring of implanted pacemakers. J Am Coll Cardiol 2009;54(22): 2012–9.

63. Mabo P, Victor F, Bazin P, et al. A randomized trial of long-term remote monitoring of pacemaker recipients (the COMPAS trial). Eur Heart J 2012;33(9):1105–11.

64. Korte T, Niehaus M, Meyer O, et al. Prospective evaluation of catheter ablation in patients with implantable cardioverter defibrillators and multiple inappropriate ICD therapies due to atrial fibrillation and type I atrial flutter. Pacing Clin Electrophysiol 2001;24(7):1061–6.

65. Miyazaki S, Taniguchi H, Kusa S, et al. Catheter ablation of atrial tachyarrhythmias causing inappropriate implantable cardioverter-defibrillator shocks. Europace 2015;17:289–94.

66. Reddy VY, Reynolds MR, Neuzil P, et al. Prophylactic catheter ablation for the prevention of defibrillator therapy. N Engl J Med 2007;357(26):2657–65.

67. Daubert JP, Zareba W, Cannom DS, et al. Inappropriate implantable cardioverter-defibrillator shocks in MADIT II: frequency, mechanisms, predictors, and survival impact. J Am Coll Cardiol 2008;51(14):1357–65.

68. Poole JE, Johnson GW, Hellkamp AS, et al. Prognostic importance of defibrillator shocks in patients with heart failure. N Engl J Med 2008;359(10): 1009–17.

69. Shukla HH, Flaker GC, Hellkamp AS, et al. Clinical and quality of life comparison of accelerometer, piezoelectric crystal, and blended sensors in DDDR-paced

patients with sinus node dysfunction in the mode selection trial (MOST). Pacing Clin Electrophysiol 2005;28(8):762–70.

70. Cole CR, Jensen DN, Cho Y, et al. Correlation of impedance minute ventilation with measured minute ventilation in a rate responsive pacemaker. Pacing Clin Electrophysiol 2001;24(6):989–93.

71. Osswald S, Cron T, Grädel C, et al. Closed-loop stimulation using intracardiac impedance as a sensor principle: correlation of right ventricular dP/dtmax and intracardiac impedance during dobutamine stress test. Pacing Clin Electrophysiol 2000;23(10 Pt 1):1502–8.

72. Proietti R, Manzoni G, Di Biase L, et al. Closed loop stimulation is effective in improving heart rate and blood pressure response to mental stress: report of a single-chamber pacemaker study in patients with chronotropic incompetent atrial fibrillation. Pacing Clin Electrophysiol 2012;35(8):990–8.

73. Whellan DJ, Droogan CJ, Fitzpatrick J, et al. Change in intrathoracic impedance measures during acute decompensated heart failure admission: results from the Diagnostic Data for Discharge in Heart Failure Patients (3D-HF) Pilot Study. J Card Fail 2012;18(2):107–12.

74. Conraads VM, Tavazzi L, Santini M, et al. Sensitivity and positive predictive value of implantable intrathoracic impedance monitoring as a predictor of heart failure hospitalizations: the SENSE-HF trial. Eur Heart J 2011;32(18):2266–73.

75. Heist EK, Herre JM, Binkley PF, et al. Analysis of Different Device-Based Intrathoracic Impedance Vectors for Detection of Heart Failure Events (from the Detect Fluid Early from Intrathoracic Impedance Monitoring Study). Am J Cardiol 2014;114(8):1249–56.

76. Bourge RC, Abraham WT, Adamson PB, et al. Randomized controlled trial of an implantable continuous hemodynamic monitor in patients with advanced heart failure: the COMPASS-HF study. J Am Coll Cardiol 2008;51(11):1073–9.

77. Abraham WT, Adamson PB, Bourge RC, et al. Wireless pulmonary artery haemodynamic monitoring in chronic heart failure: a randomised controlled trial. Lancet 2011;377(9766):658–66.

78. Ritzema J, Troughton R, Melton I, et al, Hemodynamically Guided Home Self-Therapy in Severe Heart Failure Patients (HOMEOSTASIS) Study Group. Physician-directed patient self-management of left atrial pressure in advanced chronic heart failure. Circulation 2010;121(9):1086–95.

79. Abraham WT. Disease management: remote monitoring in heart failure patients with implantable defibrillators, resynchronization devices, and haemodynamic monitors. Europace 2013;15(Suppl 1):i40–6.

80. Gibson MC, Krucoff M, Fischell D, et al. Rationale and design of the AngeLmed for Early Recognition and Treatment of STEMI trial: a randomized, prospective clinical investigation. Am Heart J 2014;168(2):168–74.

81. Guédon-Moreau L, Lacroix D, Sadoul N, et al. Costs of remote monitoring vs. ambulatory follow-ups of implanted cardioverter defibrillators in the randomized ECOST study. Europace 2014;16(8):1181–8.

82. Calò L, Gargaro A, De Ruvo E, et al. Economic impact of remote monitoring on ordinary follow-up of implantable cardioverter defibrillators as compared with conventional in-hospital visits. A single-center prospective and randomized study. J Interv Card Electrophysiol 2013;37(1):69–78.

83. Akar JG, Bao H, Jones P, et al. Use of remote monitoring of newly implanted cardioverter-defibrillators: insights from the patient related determinants of ICD remote monitoring (PREDICT RM) study. Circulation 2013;128(22):2372–83.

84. Green BB, Cook AJ, Ralston JD, et al. Effectiveness of home blood pressure monitoring, Web communication, and pharmacist care on hypertension control: a randomized controlled trial. JAMA 2008;299(24):2857–67.

85. Margolis KL, Asche SE, Bergdall AR, et al. Effect of home blood pressure telemonitoring and pharmacist management on blood pressure control: a cluster randomized clinical trial. JAMA 2013;310(1):46–56.

86. Sivakumaran D, Earle KA. Telemonitoring: use in the management of hypertension. Vasc Health Risk Manag 2014;10:217–24.

87. Shane-McWhorter L, Lenert L, Petersen M, et al. The Utah Remote Monitoring Project: improving health care one patient at a time. Diabetes Technol Ther 2014;16:653–60.

88. Cleland JG, Louis AA, Rigby AS, et al. Noninvasive home telemonitoring for patients with heart failure at high risk of recurrent admission and death: the Trans-European Network-Home- Care Management System (TEN-HMS) study. J Am Coll Cardiol 2005;45(10):1654–64.

89. Grancelli HO, Ferrante DC. Telephone interventions for disease management in heart failure. BMJ 2007;334(7600):910–1.

90. Pandor A, Gomersall T, Stevens JW, et al. Remote monitoring after recent hospital discharge in patients with heart failure: a systematic review and network meta-analysis. Heart 2013;99(23):1717–26.

91. Thokala P, Baalbaki H, Brennan A, et al. Telemonitoring after discharge from hospital with heart failure: cost-effectiveness modeling of alternative service designs. BMJ Open 2013;3(9):e003250.

92. Checchi KD, Huybrechts KF, Avorn J, et al. Electronic medication packaging devices and medication adherence: a systematic review. JAMA 2014;312(12): 1237–47.

93. Goldstein CM, Gathright EC, Dolansky MA, et al. Randomized controlled feasibility trial of two telemedicine medication reminder systems for older adults with heart failure. J Telemed Telecare 2014;20(6):293–9.

94. Fox S, Duggan M. Pew Research Center. Mobile Health 2012. Available at: http://pewinternet.org/reports. Accessed September 6, 2014.

95. Kiselev AR, Gridnev VI, Shvartz VA, et al. Active ambulatory care management supported by short message services and mobile phone technology in patients with arterial hypertension. J Am Soc Hypertens 2012;6(5):346–55.

96. Siopis G, Chey T, Allman-Farinelli M. A systematic review and meta-analysis of interventions for weight management using text messaging. J Hum Nutr Diet 2015;28(Suppl 2):1–15.

97. Rodgers A, Corbett T, Bramley D, et al. Do u smoke after txt? Results of a randomised trial of smoking cessation using mobile phone text messaging. Tob Control 2005;14(4):255–61.

98. Haug S, Schaub MP, Venzin V, et al. Efficacy of a text message-based smoking cessation intervention for young people: a cluster randomized controlled trial. J Med Internet Res 2013;15(8):e171.

99. Banchs JE, Benvenuto V, Baquero GA, et al. High adoption rates of mobile technology by cardiology clinic patients but limited use of health applications. J Am Coll Cardiol 2014;63(12_S).

100. Kwon S, Kim H, Park KS. Validation of heart rate extraction using video imaging on a built-in camera system of a smartphone. Conf Proc IEEE Eng Med Biol Soc 2012;2012:2174–7.

101. Nam Y, Lee J, Chon KH. Respiratory rate estimation from the built-in cameras of smartphones and tablets. Ann Biomed Eng 2014;42(4):885–98.

102. McManus DD, Lee J, Maitas O, et al. A novel application for the detection of an irregular pulse using an iPhone 4S in patients with atrial fibrillation. Heart Rhythm 2013;10(3):315–9.

103. Saxon LA. Ubiquitous wireless ECG recording: a powerful tool physicians should embrace. J Cardiovasc Electrophysiol 2013;24(4):480–3.

104. FDA K140933 August 15, 2014. Available at: www.fda.gov: http://google2.fda.gov/search?q=cache:RzMwCs89soAJ:www.accessdata.fda.gov/cdrh_docs/pdf14/k140933.pdf+alivecor&client=FDAgov&site=FDAgov&lr=&proxystylesheet=FDAgov&output=xml_no_dtd&ie=UTF-8&access=p&oe=UTF-8. Accessed September 6, 2014.

105. Saur NM, England MR, Menzie W, et al. Accuracy of a novel noninvasive transdermal continuous glucose monitor in critically ill patients. J Diabetes Sci Technol 2014;8(5):945–50.

106. Reynolds EM, Grujovski A, Wright T, et al. Utilization of robotic "remote presence" technology within North American intensive care units. Telemed J E Health 2012;18(7):507–15.

Index

Note: Page numbers of article titles are in **boldface** type.

A

Med Clin N Am 99 (2015) 897–912
http://dx.doi.org/10.1016/S0025-7125(15)00082-6
0025-7125/15/$ – see front matter © 2015 Elsevier Inc. All rights reserved.

medical.theclinics.com

Printed and bound by CPI Group (UK) Ltd, Croydon, CR0 4YY

22/10/2024

01777783-0001